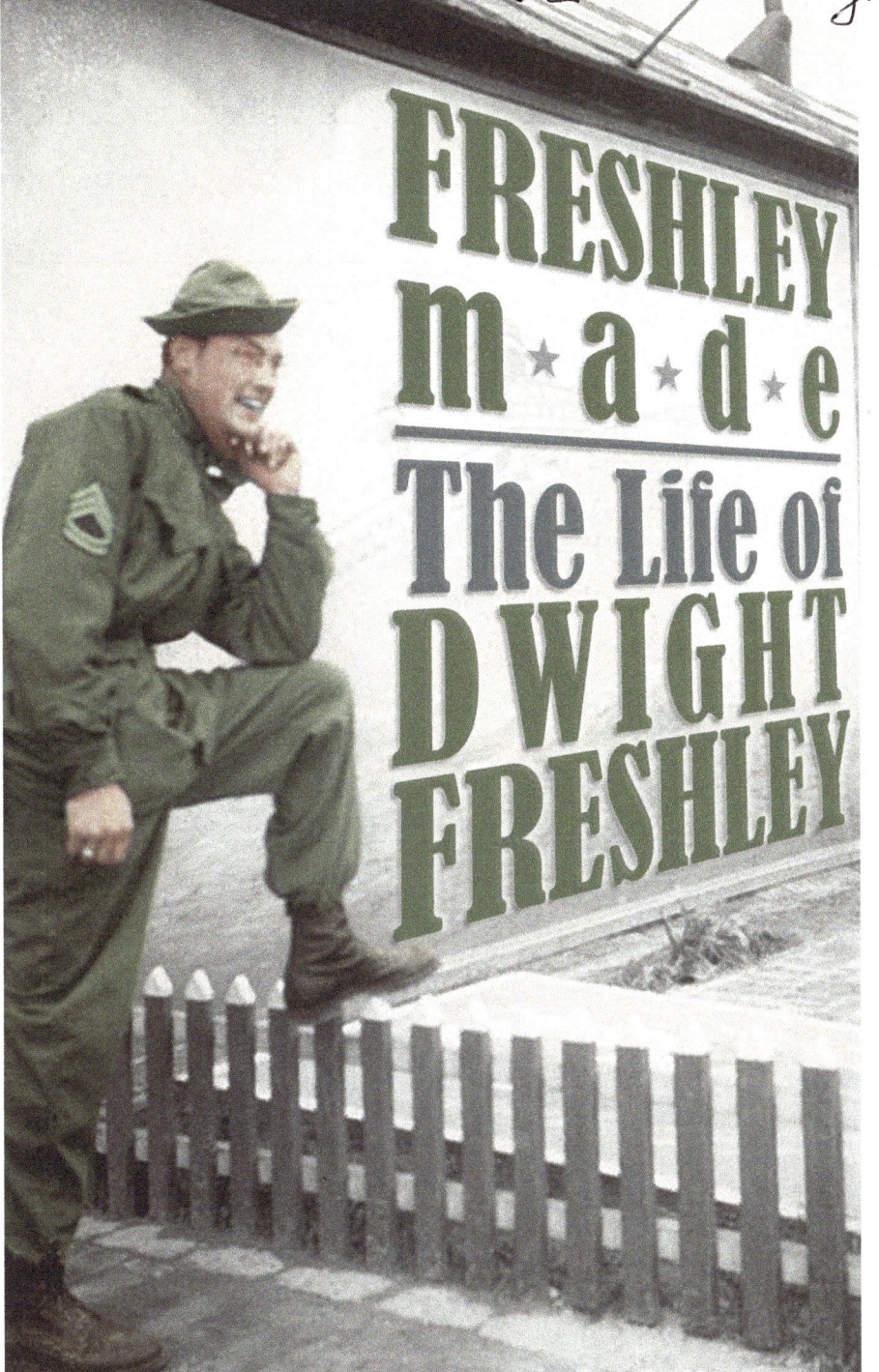

FRESHLEY m*a*d*e
The Life of DWIGHT FRESHLEY

Freshley Made:
The Life of Dwight Freshley

Copyright© 2020 by Dwight Freshely

Design Copyright© 2020 by Burns Studio Art

All rights reserved. No part of this book may be used or reproduced by any means, graphic, electronic, or mechanical including photocopying, recording, tape or by any information storage retrieval system without the written permission of the publisher except in the case of brief quotations embodied in critical articles and reviews.

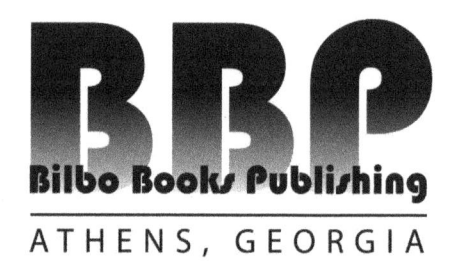

Bilbo Books Publishing
ATHENS, GEORGIA

Bilbo Books Publishing
www.BilboBooks.com

ISBN- 978-1-7326180-6-0
ISBN- 1-7326180-6-2

Printed in the United States of America

All rights reserved. Published in the United States of America by Bilbo Books Publishing. Athens, Georgia

Dedication

This book is dedicated to Jean, my partner of 63 years and my four children: Philip, Bruce, Doug and Dina. Also, I am one of seven children of Palmer and Dora. Over my life, I have been supported by my parents, brothers and sister and their spouses, and my dozens of nieces and nephews. Family has blessed and informed my thinking. I have learned you are not what you think you are…but what you think, you are.

FRESHLEY MADE:
The Life of Dwight Freshley

I have lived for ninety-five years by this point, and not to be immodest, but I've done it right. Thinking back on it, mine has been a quintessentially American life. I was born on a farm. I played in a family band in the dancehalls of Middle America in the Big Band Era. I snuck away from my father's farm to join the Army. I was sent overseas and participated in D-Day, one of those days which will live in infamy…for the Nazis. I came home and went to college. Then I went to more college. Then some more. I coached a debate team. I taught Speech Communications. I married a caring and beautiful woman. I had four kids. I had a lawn, a mortgage, all of the trappings of the standard American family. Now I'm combing through the events of my long and varied life, writing my memoirs while sitting at an assisted-living facility in Athens, Georgia.

My hearing isn't all that good. War wound…sort of. Keep reading. I'll get to it. My hearing may not be great, but my memory is outstanding. I remember my childhood movie theater in rural Ohio. I remember the make-believe games I used to play with my best friend, Dale. I remember my induction into the military. I remember subduing a would-be mugger who interrupted what should have been a solid night of collegiate necking. I remember talking to a crazy man trying to sell a crazy book on a decidedly-less-than-crazy college recruiting trip in rural South Dakota. I remember meeting my wife. I remember seeing my children for the first time. I remember people, places, events, awards, firsts and lasts, hellos and farewells, triumphs and tragedies. Mainly I remember the women…

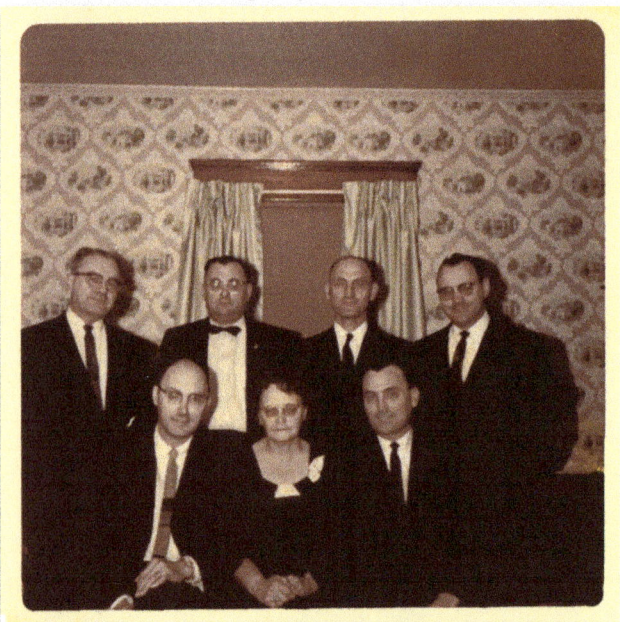

Early Days

FARM LIVING ISN'T THE LIFE FOR ME, BUT AT THAT TIME I DIDN'T GET A SAY IN THE MATTER

As many of us were back then, I was delivered into this world at home. My deliverer was my Uncle "Doc" Warren, my Mother, Dora Ann's, brother. Doc Warren's prescription for good health was simple, "Keep your bowels open and your mouth shut." A good, simple Midwestern man and a physician to boot, Uncle Doc was a star within the Freshley family.

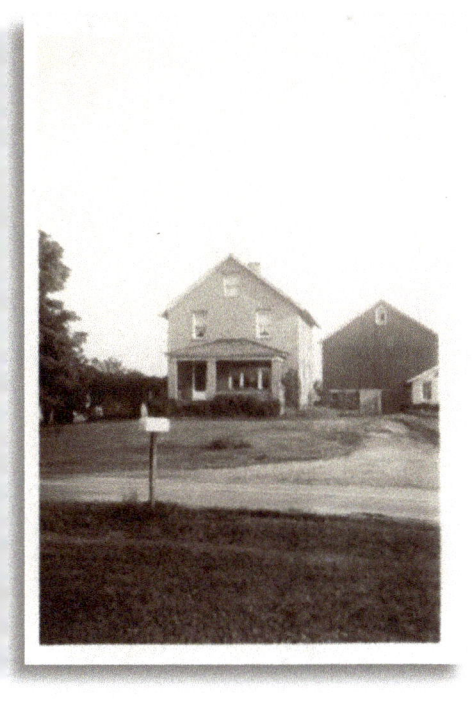

The "Home" in which I was delivered into this world was a working farm in the little, rural Midwestern town of Homeworth, Ohio, a homely farm village not too far from Akron, in the northeast corner of The Buckeye State. My family were farmers by trade and musicians by the grace of God…well God and my big sister, Ruthie.

My parents, Palmer and Dora Ann Freshley, finally closed up the baby shop when I, their seventh child, was born. I was told that on the day I was born there was a cyclone in northwest Ohio, around Lima or Toledo. I like to think of it as an omen, a good omen, but I'm a dreamer and dreamers dream.

My father Palmer Freshley was a strict but generous man. If someone nearby had a car problem, he would always take his horse and pull the car out of the ditch. But, when someone

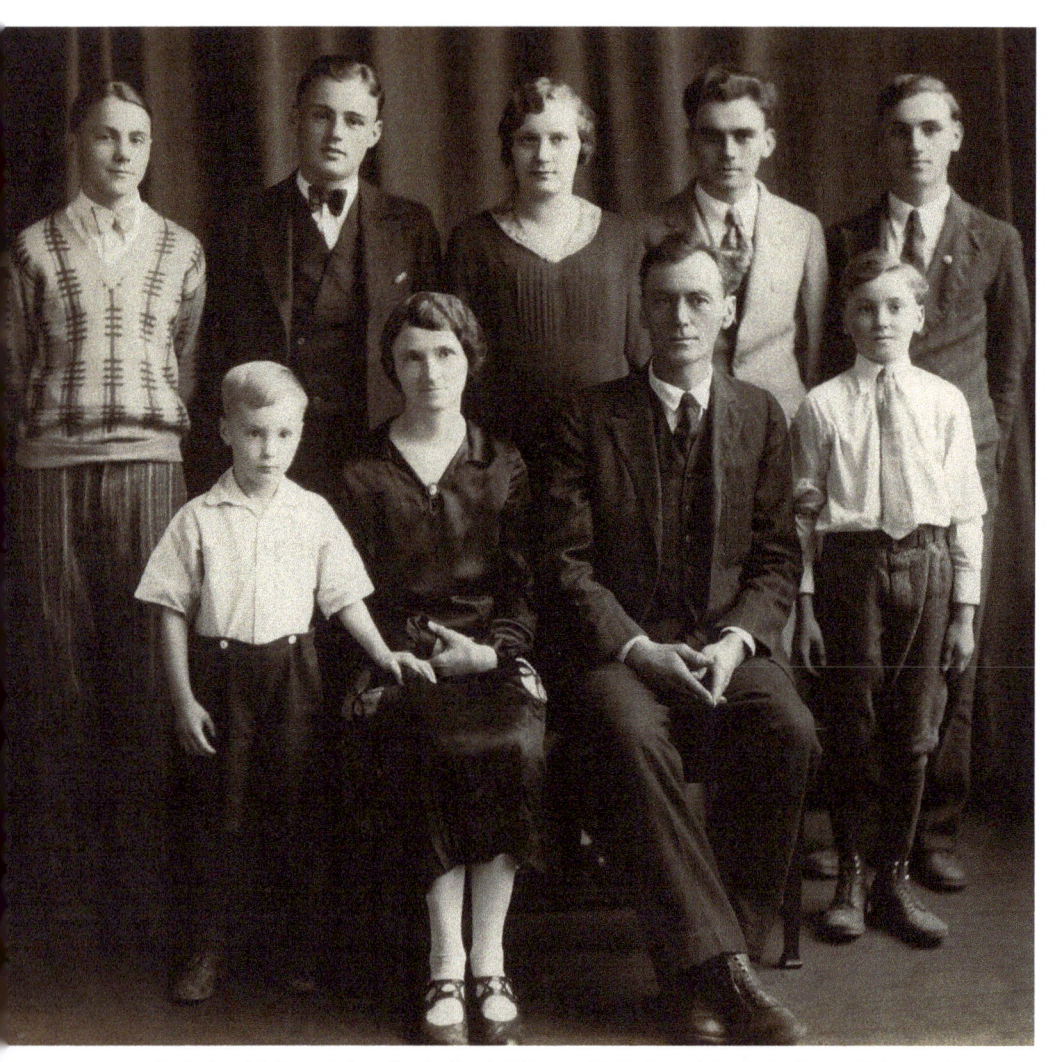

(L-R, Back) Don, Atlee, Ruth, Paul, Wilson; (L-R, Front) Dwight, Dora, Palmer, Wendell

pulled him out of the ditch, Dad would insist on paying the man. Palmer Freshley was authoritarian, often "licking me" with a stick. Dad was representative of men of his era: prideful, hard-working, fundamentally decent and disdainful of charity when it was directed at him, but generous when he was the one acting charitably.

Palmer Freshley was the oldest son of Jesse and Symonette Freshley. Aunt Edith was the second oldest…then John, then Monroe, then Edgar, then Owen, then Allen and finally Ellen. We Freshleys have never done anything halfway. When we procreate, we do it farm-style, heartily and honestly, making sure that we generate enough free child labor to keep the farm going for another generation. Farming is not an easy life, but it can be a fulfilling life. We avoided many of the pitfalls of the family farm by diversifying our family income long before it became popular. We bottled and sold milk and ice cream to our neighbors. We had a family band/orchestra, playing for local dances and events. I delivered newspapers on Saturdays. It was this diversification and entrepreneurial spirit which got us through The Great Depression in better shape than most. To be honest, we didn't even know there was a Depression.

My paternal grandfather Jesse lived in Homeworth during his retirement, in a house up on a hill overlooking town, next to a feed mill, the perfect vantage point for overseeing a farming community. Aunt Edith lived with them, and I often stopped in for a quick chat with her while on my delivery route.

My Aunt Edith was a widow who, in grand small town widow tradition, knew everybody's business. She kept me up to date with the latest gossip. Another uncle of mine ran a store downtown around the Turn of the Century. I think he sold out to Sam Herren. The other store in Homeworth belonged to the

Emmons – Harold, his wife Bessie and their son Howard. We delivered milk to both stores, conveniently located just a block apart in metropolitan downtown Homeworth. Frequently, I would get penny candy from them both.

Mother was the light of my life. She was winsome, sweet, and a tireless worker. Oh, how I looked forward to her letters when I was in the Service, for the 2&½ years I was in college, and the five years I was in graduate school (1946-51).

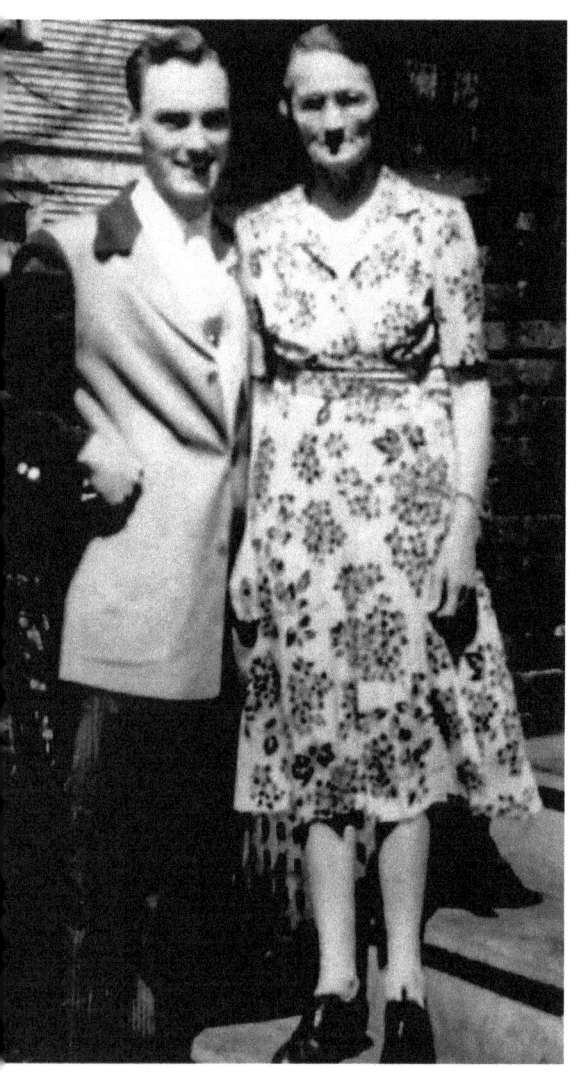

My siblings included: Ruth Alleyne (born 1907), Donald Earl (1909), Atlee Pomerene (1911), Wilson Bryan (1914), Wendell Wayne (1915), and Paul Wade (1920). I was the youngest.

My earliest youthful memory comes from a black and white photo of me, desperately trying to keep three balloons in the air. I associate this image with the visits of "The Cleveland Folks." We had cousins scattered all around. The ones we were closest to lived in the industrial, often maligned, actual metropolis of Cleveland, the industrial city which, years later, would become infamous for the time its river caught fire. The trips to see the "Cleveland Folks" were always memo-

10

rable. I distinctly remember the one trip where we struck a cow in the road with our car. I never found out how badly that cow was hurt, but I know it put a large dent in the right rear door of the Buick. I've always wondered if the cow survived. If she did, that night at milking time, I'll bet she gave a good milkshake.

On another, later, visit with the "Cleveland Folks," when I was a teenager, when we greeted our hosts, I gave my Aunt Mary a big hug. She recoiled a bit, exclaiming, "Who are you?" Ahh, family.

Somehow I recall stopping on the way back from one of those Cleveland trip to see the movie, "Little Lord Fauntleroy" with the actor Freddie Bartholomew. It's strange what one remembers, isn't it?

I remember once the "Cleveland Folks" even made a trip down to Homeworth to visit Aunt Anne & Cousin Belle, but it must not have been too exciting since I remember no actual details.

Mother's brother, Charlie Unger, lived about 300 yards down the road from us. Years later, when I could legally drive, I took him on a day of errands — all day. When I let him out of the car he handed me a dollar bill, "for your trouble." I'm not entirely sure he remembered that I was his nephew, but at least I made some money.

In family conflicts/arguments, especially those involving my malcontent brother Atlee, we tried to minimize our bad behavior for Mother's sake. Mother doted on Atlee, and we always went out of our way in order to keep Mother happy. So, even when Atlee said something rude or wildly obnoxious at the dinner table, none of us ever said a word. Because Atlee and Ruth clashed, Atlee was the one and only sibling who never played with the Freshley Family Orchestra. (In case you haven't figured it out yet, Atlee clashed with many people. He was a genius and an incredible teacher, but that didn't make him any less of a malcontent.)

The Freshly Family Orchestra played at local dances from 1933-36. We mainly performed at a dancehall named Guthrie's, but also venues at Lake Placentia, Sevekeen Lake, and Branch Range. My oldest sister Ruth was the director & custodian of the music. She was the "keeper of the precious sheet music," another reminder that she was in charge, not that we needed reminding. Ruthie was a professional piano teacher, and so, naturally, she played piano in the family band. She had 18 or 20 piano pupils and was married to a man named Wade Hoover. He went by the nickname "Dutch" and could usually be found smoking a pipe. Dutch was the patient husband, sitting to the side while Ruth directed the band, kept track of the music and taught piano lessons. Ruth was not an affectionate sister, so, it may come as a shock when I reveal that I once took her to a rendezvous with a man whom she knew growing up. They spent 15-20 minutes together. Innocent fun! At least I *think* it was innocent.

I much regret not having kept up with playing piano under Ruth's guidance. I recall we used the Vincent Lopez book of instruction. Instead of practicing something that might come in handy down the road, I was busy throwing a tennis or golf ball up against our yellow brick house (and catching it in a baseball mitt), aiming for the imaginary batter's box I had drawn on the brick wall.

Though I tried, in my way, I could not avoid the Freshley Family Orchestra. It was a part of who I was, who I am, and who I will always be. For the first three years of our existence, I wasn't a part of the orchestra, until I was old enough to join the band, replacing the one non-Freshley band member, the drummer "Brownie." When I did join the band, due to my tender age, I was treated as a sort of a Michael Jackson figure in our orchestra, a musician keeping the beat, but also a kind

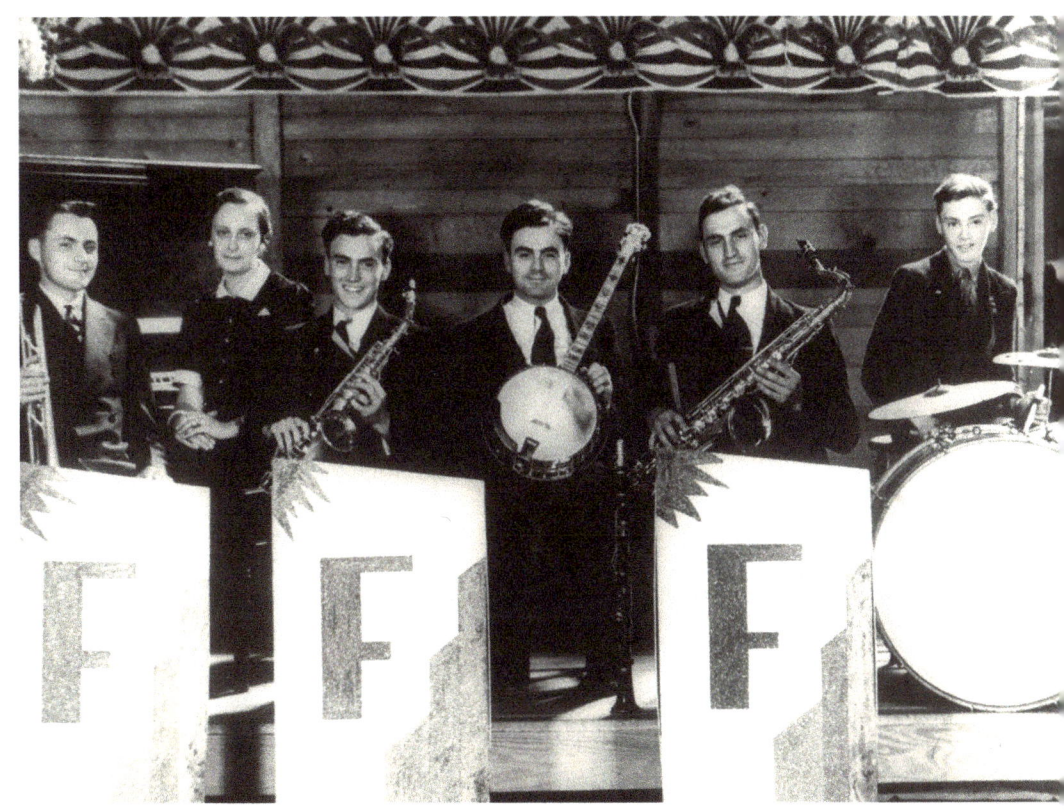

Freshley Family Orchestra, Circa 1930s: (L-R) Wendell, Ruth, Paul, Don, Wilson, Dwight

of mascot. The Freshley Family Orchestra was the accompanist to a generation of rural Ohio dancers, playing the popular songs of the era, always leaving them wanting more.

I spent a good deal, perhaps too much, of my childhood leisure time in sports. Of course my first priority other than school had to be working on the farm: hauling hay with horses, milking cows twice a day (morning and evening), keeping the hay mow in working order, and other standard farm chores.

But when I could carve out some free time, I played ball

with my buddy Dale in the pasture on the side of his house. He lived about a mile away. Dale and I devised elaborate rules, for balls, strikes, hits and outs. Like so many other imaginative American boys, we were "big leaguers"...even if only in our minds, coming from behind in the bottom of the ninth to win the day for the great state of Ohio. The Cleveland Indians were the closest professional team, and so, naturally I was a big time Indians fan.

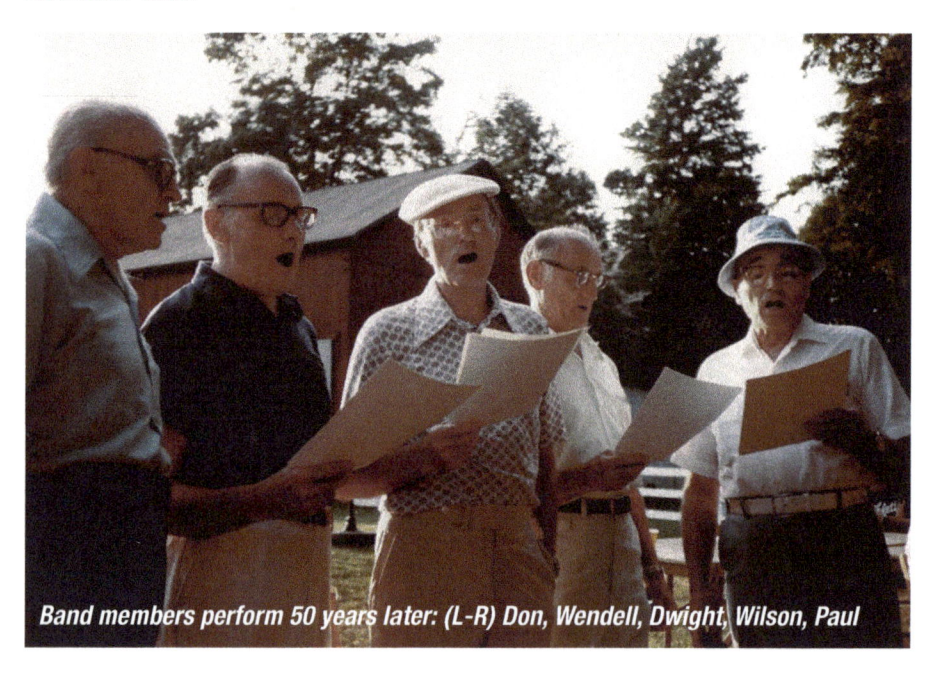

Band members perform 50 years later: (L-R) Don, Wendell, Dwight, Wilson, Paul

On Saturday nights I went to town with Dale and his family, a weekend activity which the Thomases did regularly. Dale and I would be in the backseat, watching enraptured as his father would inevitably start "feeling up" his wife's legs. That prompted Dale and me to explore our own genitals. Dale and I would leave the Thomases to their grown-up activities and wander over to The Strand heater to see a cowboy movie with Tom Mix, Bob Steele, or the Lone Ranger.

Curiously, I don't recall double dating with Dale and his steady in high school, because we weren't as close then as we had been as young boys. Friends drift apart. It happens. I do recall that Dale died first, many years later of course. I remember visiting his wife, whose name just flew out the window (I hope it returns.). We went our separate ways before arriving at Alliance High School. I got it into high school gear and Dale hardly got started.

Let's pause for a dog story. The Thomases had a hound dog which I must have petted inside their house many times, but never outside. Despite his apparent affection, that dog was moodier than I thought. One Sunday afternoon when I walked down their sidewalk, the hound was lying in front of the back door, which visitors had to climb to get to their stoop. I negotiated the first steps OK, but then I brought my right foot to the top step. The hound plunged his teeth into my right instep, ripping my flesh asunder. Guy Thomas, Dale's Dad, took me up to Uncle Doc Warren's office and we met him there that Sunday afternoon. (There were no Emergency Rooms then.) And Uncle Doc sewed me up with six stitches. I don't think he charged a dime. Ahh, family connections. I carry that scar to this day.

In addition to exercising my pitching arm, I also exercised my non-sporting imagination as a child. Around age 12 or 14, I vividly remember writing two stories. One was patterned after the, then-popular, Frank Merriwell comic book series: Merriwell was always the hero I could relate to. The second was the story of two young adventurous boys, Chip Collins and Stan Kent, who lived in an Ohio town we'll call Hudson, Ohio.

Chip and Stan were the brave and dashing heroes of the adventurous mystery stories I created around them. Of course, these two "fictional" characters were carbon copies of my pal, Dale, and me, but that's where fiction usually begins. The central character would always face an "evil" adversary and perform some heroic act to solve the problem.

The family band was work, but fun work. As I've mentioned, our main orchestral performance venue was Guthrie's, owned, as you might guess, by the Guthrie family. They had a daughter named Ruth who was sweet on my brother Paul. Her friend Sarah doted on Wendell. They would fraternize for a few minutes during Intermission. Six months later Paul and

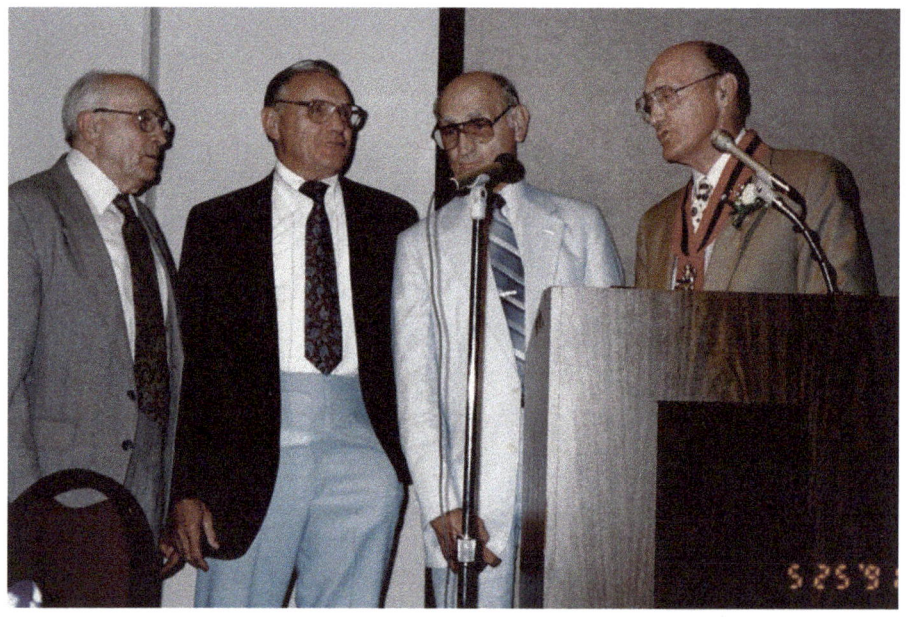

Family Reunion performance of surviving brothers in 90s: (L-R) Paul, Wendell, Wilson, Dwight

Wendell were reflecting on the girls, when Wendy (Wendell) asked Paul, "Hey, how's Ruthie?" Paul said, "Great. You know, just like Ginger Rogers, she does what Fred Astaire does backwards. She's also a sweet person."

Paul asked Wendell, "How's Sarah?" Wendell replied, "Well, she can't dance, but boy can she Intermission!"

Another dance hall we played was Silver Fox. Dad was adamantly against our playing at a venue which sold beer, but he relented a bit on the Silver Fox because the bar was separate from the dance hall. Methinks my father was splitting hairs, but he was so enamored of his kids' playing that I'm sure he overlooked some things.

I should introduce the family players: Ruth on piano, Don on banjo, Wilson on B flat Alto saxophone, Wendell on trumpet, Paul on E-Flat sax (1932-36) and drums (1932-35), "Brownie" on drums (1935-36). Brownie's replacement was better known as Dwight, or better yet, me. The money we made helped put my brother Wilson through two years of college at Kent State. Atlee would have played trombone with us if he could have gotten along with his sister. He was talented on the horns, but alas, he never made the effort to be fraternal enough for Ruthie to allow him to play with us.

In the years before I replaced Brownie played, I stayed home with Mother and sold ice cream from our basement while my siblings were entertaining the neighbors. People drove 20 miles to get our Freshley Fresh Ice Cream. And why wouldn't they? It was made with 4.7 ounces of butter fat. Why we didn't all die of a fat-induced heart attack, I'll never know. FREOK, so I do have four stents in my heart, but other than that I'm fine.

Education

When my progeny read this, they will smile as they remember my telling them how their daddy had to wade arduously though four-foot snow drifts, walking the near mile to the little red brick schoolhouse in Homeworth. I repeated this practice (up hill both ways of course) through eighth grade.

My elementary school was a classic small-town, two-room structure with grades 1-4 on the first floor and grades 5-8 on the second. Recalling the 3rd and 4th grades with the beautiful Miss Stoffer, I recall my intense crush on her. I idolized her to the extent that I couldn't fantasize about my being with her, instead imagining that she was married to a sports hero of mine, the great baseball pitcher of that time and place, Willie Shopfer. I had seen him pitch at Lake Placentia, and in my mind the hero pitcher simply had to have a lovely cheerleader, and there was no one lovelier than Miss Stoffer. It rarely happened outside of my head, but it did begin a life full of wondrous fantasy. In 4th grade I had a seat where I could lean against the chimney and hide my hand while it discreetly held the adorable hand of the red-headed Martha Pilmer, who sat directly in front of me.

Fifth and sixth grade included a promotion to the upstairs floor, a big deal when you're 11-years-old. Mr. Melvin York, the infamous eraser throwing educator, was my fifth grade teacher. When students misbehaved Mr. York would haul off and send a missile zooming at them. His pinpoint aim regularly stopped us in our tracks. I was his target once. That day,

I was seated at my desk with a pencil leaning against my forehead, not completely paying attention, until Mr. York's eraser jolted me back to reality. Luckily he didn't hit the pencil, as

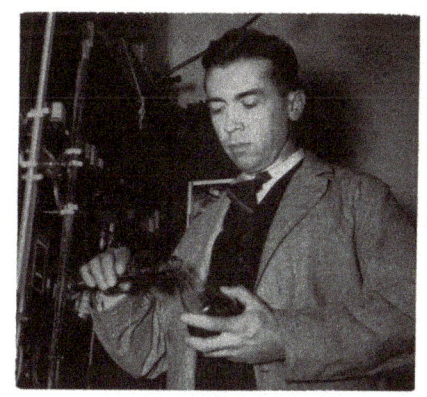

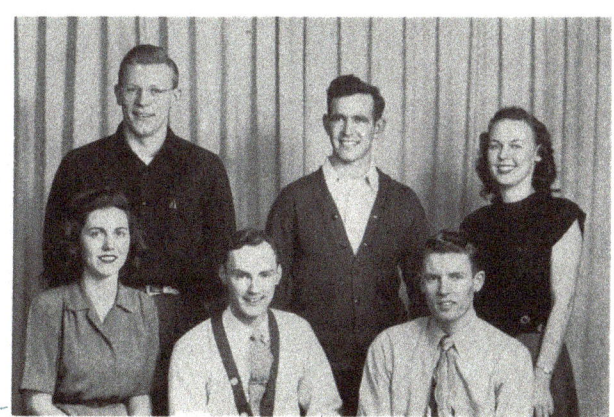

DR. KOTEN

Class of
'50

We, too, make our bid for distinction. We have power: witness the two victories in the tug of war, the traditional underclass battle, where the present juniors and freshmen suffered muddy clothes and injured pride. We have size. Aren't we the largest aggregation ever to sit in a North Central Chapel? Weren't we the largest entering class in the history of the school? We have ability. Sophomores play on all the varsity athletic teams. Every campus organization is fortunate to have our class members as their own members. The Sophomore talent show was a success. We have looks. The girls of the class of '50 are the best looking in school this year. We have ideals. We intend to continue our work at college to make our class the most outstanding in the history of the school. The juniors will get the feast of their lives next year when we offer them the banquet that is customary. Perhaps they will be able to lose sight of that terrific defeat we gave them on the banks of the old DuPage.

CLASS OFFICERS

President
 D. FRESHLEY

Vice-President
 L. ANDERSON

Treasurer
 J. KENNAUGH

Secretary
 J. RINEHART

Women's Representative
 M. LUTZ

Men's Representative
 J. BERGER

19

close to my eye as it was, or there could have been quite a lawsuit (though we were not the litigious society we are now) and I'd be nearly blind as well as nearly deaf.

My other lasting memory from that year was much more pleasant and centered around Mr. York's golden-haired, freckle-faced daughter, whose skill at eraser-tossing might not have been on par with her father's, but she knew how to hit a dead center bullseye in her own way. The Yorks lived in nearby Valley, Ohio, so she didn't attend school with me, but when there was a PTA meeting I would tag along, hoping to interact with the exotic Valley beauty. Sadly, I never had a date with her when we reached high school.

Sixth grade brought me under the tutelage of the fox-faced Mr. Walton. (No offense intended to Mr. Walton or to foxes in general, but the man's thin and wily profile did suggest our wild animal friend.) He was a disciplinarian and I was always getting into mischief, so we got to know each other

---

Senior Sketch
by JACK KOTEN

FIFTY YEARS FROM NOW if anyone asks who the most outstanding member of the Class of '50 was the name most likely to be mentioned will be that of this week's senior. No other mid-century graduate has done as much for North Central as Dwight L. Freshley. Known by all as Dee, or Uncle Dee of NCC, he not only has attained the position of President of the Student Body, but also has managed to engage himself in many many campus activities. More than twenty student organizations have been fortunate enough to number him among their members.

In Dee one may find a personality who is the reflection of many moods. Best known for his quick wit and glib tongue, he also has a mellow serious side which he manages to keep hidden from most people. There is little question about Dee's capabilities. His fertile brain is forever creating new ideas which Dee hastens to put into action as soon as possible—unless his serious self warns him not to. As a leader and an organizer he is without parallel on campus. Sincerity and humbleness are two characteristics which Dee likes to stress. Sometimes he appears over-sincere and too humble.

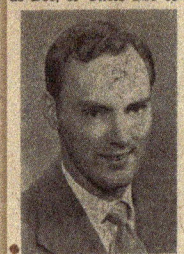

Dee Freshley

A recent example of Dee's many talents was the song he wrote and sang for the Starlite Park show. Writing lyrics and music is one of Dee's hobbies. "Ring Around the Moon" was written about two years ago when the idea for the song hit Dee. The rush for the piano was inevitable and he didn't leave until the song was completed. The title song "Yassuh" which was written for the Varsity Club's minstrel show is another example of Dee's work. Others which he has written include the "Class of '50," "I'll Never Be the Same," "Coed in the Campus," and "Don't Stop Saying I Love You." As yet Dee hasn't had any of his songs published mainly because he hasn't tried. Among the established pop songs Dee listed "Moonlight Serenade," "Star Dust," and "I'll Be Seeing You" as favorites. Les Brown's recording of "I've Got My Love To Keep Me Warm" is one of the few discs Dee owns. Dee isn't one-sided in his musical tastes however. Debussy, Tschaikowsky, and Gershwin have an ardent admirer in NCC's student body president. "Good music is a must in the well balanced life," says Dee.

MADEMOISELLE SICRE has made the deepest impression of the faculty on Dee. He has enjoyed her most because, as he says, "... of her vivacity, her spontaneity, living her philosophy of life consistently, and her genuineness." The two courses he has liked best have been philosophy of Culture and Creative Writing. With majors in English and speech, Dee will finish in June with a B.A. degree.

Twenty-two days after graduation the personable senior will reach his twenty-sixth birthday. He would like to be able to assist the *college* next year in its expanding public relations program. Student *teaching*, Dee has already a particular field which he feels he would best be suited for. Dee has already been accepted in both the University of Wisconsin's and Northwestern University's graduate schools of speech.

> "People above all else are my major interest. I believe there is much good to be derived from every personality," Dee said when queried on the subject. He has evidenced his interest in people many times during his short sojourn here at North Central. Another interest of his is banana cream pie and pork tenderloin. Aqua is his favorite color.
>
> **THIS PAST WEEK** Dee was able to witness the completion of what he calls the most thrilling moments he has seen on college athletic fields. That was when Danny Dobrowski, with a three and two count, two out in the ninth, North Central trailing 6-5 and Dick Braun raring to go on first, belted one over the right field fence to give the Cardinals a hard earned victory. The victory over Wheaton in the double overtime here, and Harry Stelling's last minute catch of a pass in the Iowa Central grid game to put the Cards out front started the cycle of thrilling last minute victories. Dee has always been interested in sports. While still quite young he set his life's ambition as becoming a big league baseball player. If he couldn't make the grade he decided he would like to become a baseball radio announcer. His constant imitation of the sportcaster who did the Cleveland Indians' home games, he believes, is one of the reasons he has developed a high nasal voice.
>
> One of the great thrills in Dee's college career occurred last College Day when he was handed the gavel by former student body president Ken Truckenbrod. "I think my greatest thrill though, while in college came when I was master of ceremonies of a show at the Shriner Crippled Children's Hospital while on deputation. I shall never forget the glistening looks in their eyes as long as I live." During Dee's two and a half years in service he was able to realize a dream that he never thought would come true. That was whistling down the main streets of New York, London, Paris, Berlin, and Rome.
>
> North Central is almost a family tradition with Dee. Two of his brothers graduated from here in 1941. Having his niece Marilyn Hoover here has been wonderful according to Dee. "Dee has been a very good uncle, but to me he's been more like a big brother," Marilyn said. Dee feels that if we "sincerely try to understand our fellow students and by being a real North Central salesman in our hometowns and keep sending high calibre students here, we can make NCC a better school."
>
> **WHAT DEE HAS LIKED BEST** about North Central has been, "The facilities to accomplish what I stated I was coming for four years ago: to grow in the four square life, physically, mentally, spiritually, and socially with the close contact with the profs highlighting it."
>
> Dee tries to be friendly with everyone. A middle-of-the-roader he would rather concede a point than do anything that would offend someone. Dee's effervescent personality comes out to meet you before a word has been said. It gives him a great appeal with the masses. Dee was president of his class for two years, a distinction seldom achieved on campus, president of the French Club, Social Committee chairman, and Homecoming co-chairman. He has been a member of the Radio Club, Honor Society, Who's Who, Pi Kappa Delta, Alpha Psi Omega, Sigma Tau Delta, Y.M.C.A. cabinet, Religious Life Council, Student Finance Board, debate team, chapel choir, glee club, and the band. He has appeared in numerous dramatic productions such as, "John Loves Mary," "Joan of Lorraine," "Macbeth," "Shake Hands With the Devil," "Abie's Irish Rose," and "Triumph in Ashes." Directing "The Family Doctor" was a great experience for Dee. Quoting Dee is the best way to sum up his complex personality. "When I'm creating something, whether a game for a party, or a friendship, I'm having a good time."

very well that year. To alter my unacceptable behavior, I was often marched out onto the landing where the stairs went down on either side. He would close the door, take off his belt and whip me. That was pretty normal in those days, but it never had the intended result. Every time he took off his belt, his pants would begin to fall down, which made me laugh, which made him mad, which made him whip me all the more,

The 7th and 8th grades were strange, largely because my brother Atlee was my teacher. Although Atlee was not an amiable person, nor a very good sibling, he was a great educator. I don't want to get too sentimental and say that he was the best elementary teacher I had, but he was. Why? First, I learned a lot. Second, he introduced me to many hobbies I otherwise would not have known and loved. We all had to pursue a hobby in 7th and 8th grade. Mine was scrap-booking. I had two themes: sports and aviation. I found dozens of pictures of airplanes and pasted them into a book, which I still have. I went wild with the sports book

— mostly football and baseball. Notre Dame had a running back then by the name of William Shakespeare. I kid you not. In the pros, the Washington Redskins had a quarterback named Sammy Baugh. I worshipped them both. My love of baseball had a bonus feature…baseball cards. I collected baseball cards, especially those which came with gum, and I had most of the "biggies": Babe Ruth, Lou Gehrig, Charley Keller, Whitlow Wyatt, Earl Averill (centerfielder for the Cleveland Indians), etc. My teacher/ brother, Atlee, was also a huge sports fan, so I guess my project went over well.

Only later did I discover another new hobby, one that would stick with me — theatre. In the seventh grade I was in a play called something like "Barnaby Bridge from Pleasant Ridge." I don't recall the name of the eighth grade play, but it opened on January 21, 1938. It was in this play that I got to have my first stage kiss: Eddie and June Bradshaw. It was a little awkward for a couple of eighth graders, but if I may offer a bit of advice for young male thespians — Anytime you're ordered to kiss a girl and you don't have to work for it, go for it.

A final innovation for a "one horse" school in the 1930's was having a formal graduation ceremony: with girls in white dresses and boys in navy blazers and white flannel trousers. The top four honor students were recognized. Those four turned out to be three girls and the teacher's brother (me). Although this honor was to reward my work for all eight years of grade school, I was still afraid that people would think I was honored because I was the teacher's brother. Maybe I was, but I was still a diligent student.

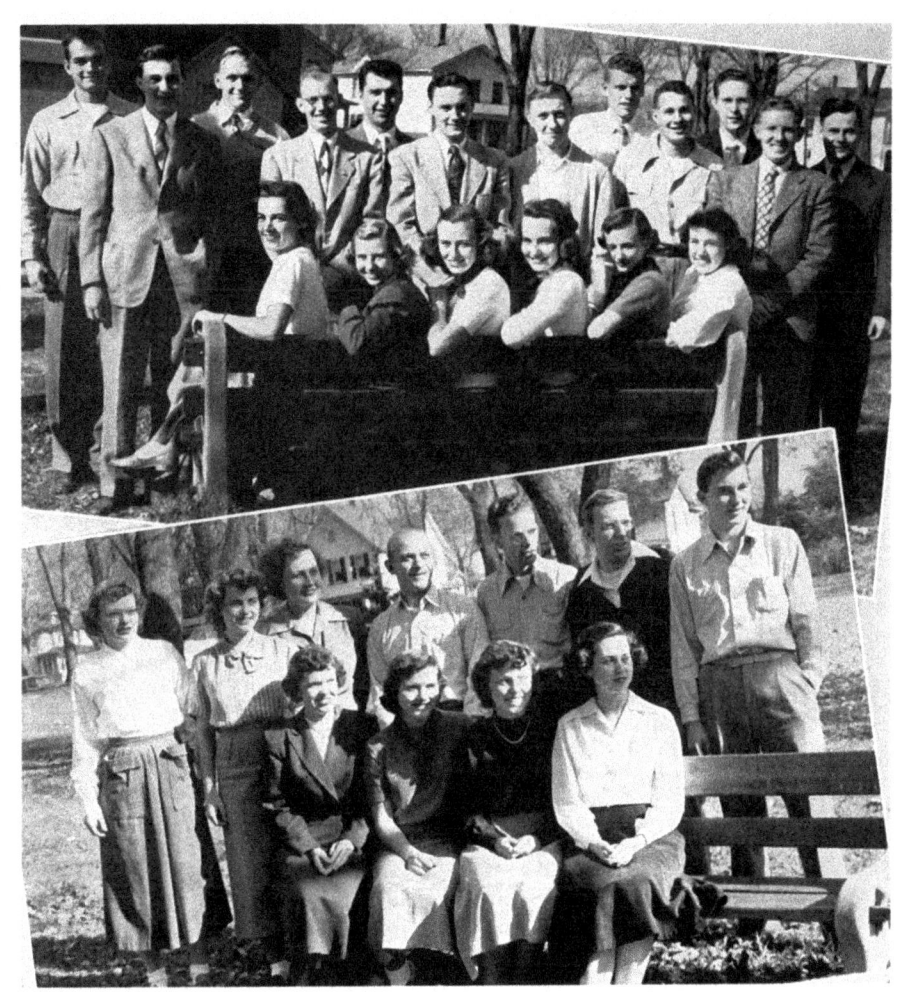

Back Row, (left to right):
Hanne, Spreng, S.monsen, J Wolf, Fenske, Freshley, Ester, Adams, Grandlienard, Bloede, G Spong, Schap
Seated, (left to right)
P Ebinger, M. Siemsen, Hoover, Norberg, Van Adestine, Eigenbrodt

Standing (left to right):
Kirn, Ritzman, Miss Hargis, Trapp, McDonald, Shilt, Spreng
Seated, (left to right):
Foster, R Johnson, Emholtz, Cameron

Student Council

"To promote a spirit never before equaled."

The gavel of the 1949-1950 Student Council opened a year of innovations in student government. Open meetings to the student body, sponsored activities, such as the Torchlight Parade, Woe Week, Homecoming, Wheaton exchanges, College Day, and all school elections. Individual interest for the bettering of N.C.C. inspired and enhanced integration of social activities, co-ordination with faculty and sincere efforts to keep the student body informed.

Social Committee

Providing North Central with such events as the Frosh Reception, Sadie Hawkins Day, the Thanksgiving Tea, and the County Fair, this able group has again shown its worth to the campus community.

Under the leadership of Rollie Trapp, student chairman, and Miss Mary Louise Hargis, faculty advisor, the Social Committee has successfully provided a wholesome and varied social life on the campus.

Work

CHILD LABOR AND OTHER PROFITABLE ENDEAVORS

My father, Palmer, ran a store in Homeworth earlier in his career. He must have moved out of town and into the house where I was born around 1910. And that house had a farm! It was a forty-acre lot, not large by today's standards but enough to sustain a twelve-cow Jersey herd. We also had an orchard full of peaches, plums and pears, and, my mother's pride and joy, a garden.

The farm boasted maple trees, from which we extracted sap for making maple syrup. There was a chestnut tree. And there was an oil well — which never made Palmer rich but did fuel some childhood fantasies. On the side of our property, there was a lane about the length of a football field leading into the woods.

One of my farm chores was to bring the cows in from the woods and the pasture. I learned to milk cows early in life, and I think Dad was always a little resentful of the fact that I could milk faster than he. When I was a teenager, he accused me of wanting to finish sooner so I "could run to town"…and, of course, he was right.

I can't recall how much farm work my oldest brothers, Don and Atlee, did. I know Wilson and Wendell ("Wendy") milked too, and worked other aspects of the farm. Wilson had a knack of always being there at the right time to help Dad and he worked hard (probably why I often referred to him, in the parlance of the times, as a "prince of a guy"). Wendy wasn't always in Dad's good graces and he was asked to leave the farm. He reported that he was "kicked off the farm," but with less anger than Atlee's booting. Let's face it, my father was an Authoritarian. If you crossed him, it would cost you. He eventually mellowed. I vividly remember, in his latter years, being at the opposite end of the dinner table and playfully asking him to "Pass the salt, Walt," and not getting taken to the woodshed.

We Freshleys had a working dairy, and peddled milk to somewhere in the range of 30-35 customers in town. We did not pasteurize our milk, instead choosing to "aerate" it, and as far as I know, not one person got sick from drinking our milk in all the years I was home. The bottles had long necks and the cream "rose to the top" of those necks. When you poured that cream over your breakfast cereal, it was heavenly. (I ate wheat cereal, especially Wheat Chex, from the Purina folks at Checkerboard Square. Once I ate enough to get an autographed picture from the cowboy-actor Tom Mix, inscribed "To my straight shooting pal, Dwight." I still have that metal framed photo.)

On those forty acres of ours we harvested hay, wheat, oats, corn and soy beans. I believe Dad was the first entrepreneurial farmer to introduce soy beans to Columbia County. It soon became prevalent on Ohio farms. There were two kinds of hay: timothy and clover. Timothy hay was more common, and clover hay was more exotic. The bees liked its blossoms much more. As I'm sure is the case with every single other child ever raised on a farm, I distinctly remember "hauling hay," using our faithful draught horses to pull the heavy hay rack. There was a slope going to the big barn doors, and there were framed, 8x8 hay mows on both sides as you drove into the barn. One day when "Wendy" and I were doing the "hay honors," and I was feeling mischievous, I snuck up to the hay mow and impishly urinated on my unsuspecting brother below. Then the chase was on — with Dwight jumping out to an early lead — angry, urine-soaked Wendy gaining steam — and finally with Dwight's losing of his footing, falling from the hay mow and cracking his collar bone.

Yet again, I woke up in Uncle Doc's office.

We had horses, many of them, but only three stand out in my memory: Barney, June and Blandy. Old Barney must've lived until he was 20. He was a sorrel horse whom Dad bought with a fistula, or running sore, on his shoulder. I do recall our vet's

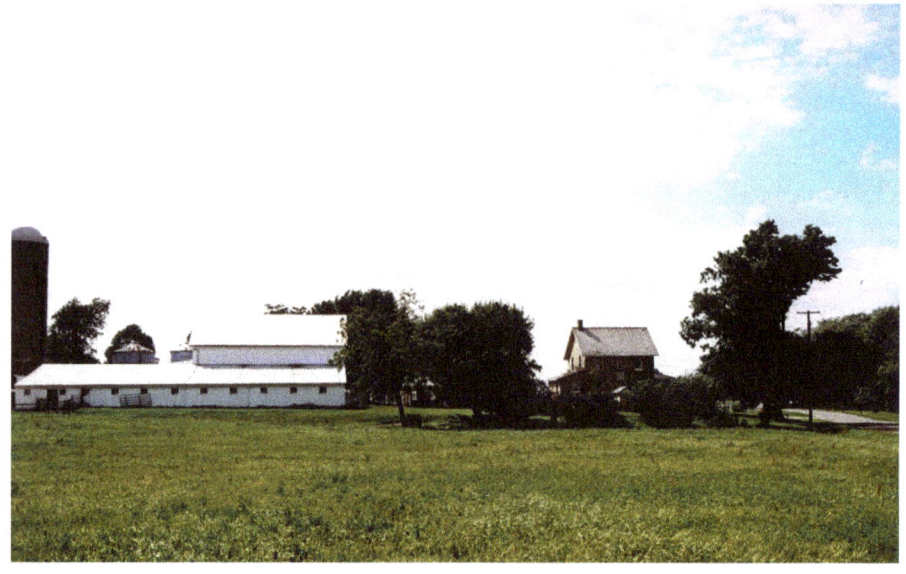

treating Barney, but I don't recall Barney's complaining one bit (a horrible horse pun I couldn't help making). With medication Barney continued to wear a collar, pull a plow, or a harrow, or, for that matter, an entire hay wagon. I developed untold affection for that horse.

June was a dappled gray, chunky like a Belgian, which was Blandy's breed. I had the thrill of riding Blandy home the day Dad bought him. I learned rudimentary sexuality at an early age from those horses. It's almost impossible not to on a farm. The fascinating thing about Blandy was that he had only one testicle. The other never descended.

Back when Dad attended Mount Union College (I never did find out how long he went), he had to turn in an expository essay, and his was on horses. The professor's evaluation? "That's the best description of a horse I have ever read." Yes, we all heard that story more times than I could count.

As I've said, we had a dairy farm with Jersey cows, and we milked, bottled, and peddled that milk to 30+ customers. After milking, I would help Mother in the basement early, and later with the bottling in the milk house. We delivered milk in at least two kinds of cars: a Model A Ford, and a 1928 Buick. Our delivery time was between 8 & 9, not 5 or 6, as was normal! When I went into the service in 1943 I received a letter from Mrs. Ditty, one of the people on our milk route, that read, "Dwight, I don't miss you, but I miss your whistling." Maybe I woke her up one too many times at 9 AM. And then there was that frigid Midwestern winter morning with dangling icicles galore when I took in Edna and Charlie Maxwell's milk, I must've bumped a huge icicle, and it came down and hit me in the forehead, requiring stitches. Uncle Doc was familiar with me by then. Dangerous business, those milk routes.

Freshley's also made homemade ice cream from that incomparable Jersey milk and cream, which people would happily drive miles to buy. As I've mentioned before, on Wednesdays and Saturday nights (before I was old enough to join the band), when the Freshley Family Orchestra was busy playing for dances, I would stay at home and help Mother sell ice cream. Ice cream never tasted better than it did on the farm. Eat your heart out, Edy's.

My eyes have never been great. My hearing is now fairly awful, too, but I can trace that development directly to an incident in the War. We'll get there in a bit. As a teen, I had a feeling that I might need glasses. But what specifically prompted me to go to the ophthalmologist was sitting in Miss Ruth Weaver's World History class, when she called on me. "Dwight, what happened on that date on the board?" I answered, "What date on the board?" She said, "Please see me after class." After class, she offered to buy glasses for me! Though my folks might not have been able to pay for them, I believe my brother, Wilson, would have helped me out. Either way, a kind and observant teacher helped me again.

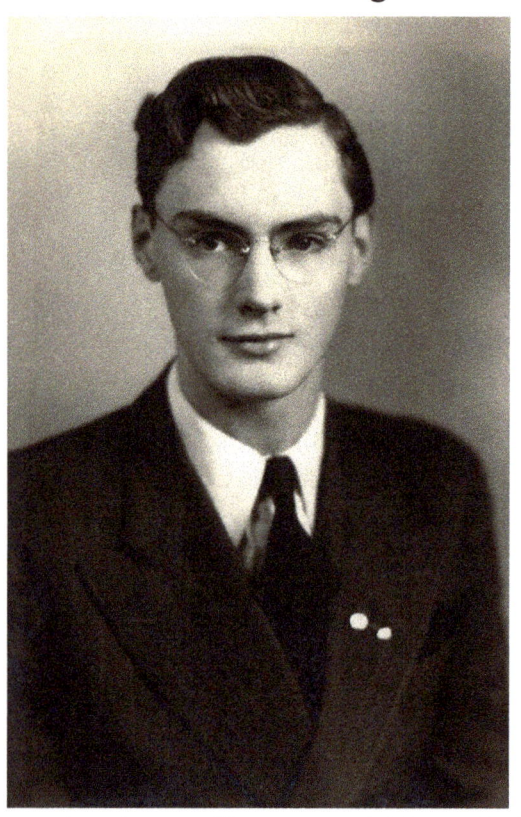

As a teenager, when I wasn't doing chores, work or homework I followed my passions. I was admittedly extremely interested in the newfound wonders of the opposite sex, but I was also a dedicated young Christian in an era of relative innocence. After attending Christian Endeavor, a weekly young people's religious meeting Sunday nights, I would always take Pearl Reed home afterward. She lived across from the train depot. WARNING! Coming up is an anecdote which may be a candidate for the Guinness Book of World Records for…cue the trumpets please…holding a kiss while 119 freight cars rolled past! You may now applaud. Thank you. Thank you all.

I really feel guilty about Pearl's and my relationship. We had a regular Sunday night date. I only went out of town one time, to a church 10-15 miles away. We piled into three cars — young, eager, theoretically Christian, teenagers sitting on each other's laps. Pearl sat on mine. I felt awkward, with no place to put my hands, so I rested them just past her knee. She half-moaned, "Please, please." I didn't know if she meant "Please stop" or "Please go ahead," so I removed my hand, never knowing the precise meaning of her pleas of "please." In retrospect, I should've asked for some clarification.

Another C.E. (Christian Endeavor) "date" was Donna Gardner, who lived directly across from the church. I may have taken her to a movie. Heads up for the summary statement:

In high school (grades 10, 11 and 12) I had 100 dates with 40 different girls.

That number may sound unbelievable to modern readers, but dating was a little different back then. It was a lot more casual, especially among teenagers. There was less (overt at least) jealousy. There was more simply enjoying each others' company. And it was less overtly focused toward marriage, at least in the boys' minds.

To add to my ever-growing list of hobbies, I rediscovered the joy of writing in high school. When I was a senior taking "Journalism," each Tuesday we would lay out the stories for the Friday edition of the Red + Blue. I had already asked fellow journalist, Julia Temple, out for a date to the school prom. She was a junior. I was a senior. On "Layout Day" she said to me, "Dwight, I want to talk to you tomorrow." I vividly recall thinking, while doing the milking that night, "She's going to break our date. But I'll just play it cool. Hey, she's not the only grain of sand on the beach." Sure enough, the next day Julia explained, "Dwight, you know Art Stanley and I are co-chairs of the Jr-Sr Prom?" You can guess how it went from there. With only the aid of my expansive imagination and a cow's sagging udders, I had guessed correctly the night before. The juniors put on the prom for the seniors, and the theme was a "Promme Militia." Students came in decorated garb under crossed swords. It was quite dramatic and memorable. Instead of Julia, I ended up taking Olive John, a senior.

Perhaps you recall that I earlier reported my summary figure of 100 dates with 40 different girls. It's just a few pages back. Feel free to turn back and look it up, I'll wait. The fact is, I did not go steady with any of them. I "played the field," as we said in those days.

This is a representative joke from the time of my childhood. It's the story of a young fellow preparing himself for a big date, going to the drug store to get some condoms. He furtively sneaks around the druggist's counter until the druggist asks, "May I help you?" The teenager hems and haws. The druggist, realizing his embarrassment, says, "Would two condoms be OK?" The boy says, "Sure, how much?" "Two dollars." The prospective Romeo pays the druggist and goes on his way.

Later that evening, after dressing to the nines and slathering on some aftershave, the young man drives to his girlfriend's house. He goes up to the door and his date's father answers the door. And guess who it is? You guessed it – it was the druggist who sold him the condoms.

My high school put on the Gilbert and Sullivan musical, "The

HMS Pinafore." I played Captain Corcoran. Suzanne William played Buttercup, singing the song "I Called Little Buttercup," suggesting the small size of the character and, presumably, the actress as well. Unfortunately for us, Sue was 5'7", and weighed in at around 120 lbs. Despite that minor discrepancy, the show was a big success.

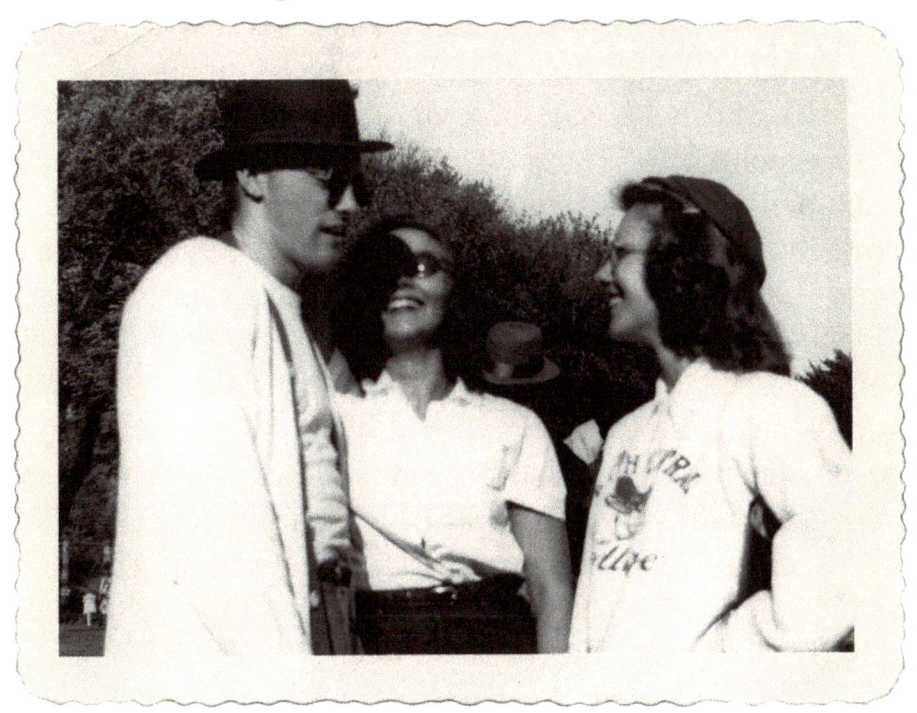

The choice of the senior play was based on the ease of casting for Miss Geddert, the Drama Director (from Hood College). There were so many beautiful girls in the class that the play pretty well had to be "Stage Door," a then-popular show about a dozen super-attractive, budding actresses living just off Broadway, all searching for their big break in front of the bright lights of The Great White Way. The real Broadway show starred Ginger Rogers and Linda Darnell, with Adolph Mangeneau playing the impresario. I played that impresario role in our production.

As a result of my drama participation, I was inducted into the National Thespian Society as well as Alpha Psi Omega for Fine Arts, even serving as president of the Thespians. Other activities included singing with the double quartet and the mixed choir. I also played the snare drum in the marching band and tympani (kettle drums) in the concert band. By far, the biggest performance thrill I had as a youngster was inaugurating the Akron (Ohio) Rubber Bowl, in the fall of 1941.

Eventually I graduated from Alliance High School. I recall Wendell's 1933 yearbook caption, "It don't mean a thing if you don't have that swing." And Harry Porter, who lived a block away from me, wrote, "All great men are dying. Hmm. Hmm. I don't feel so good myself." When it came time for mine in 1942, it read, "With memorable words of choice, he could move thousands with his voice." I did have a pretty good voice, and became an accomplished speaker, later pursuing a career as a professor of Speech Communications.

My yearbook would record that I graduated twelfth out of 220 seniors. I was asked to speak at the Baccalaureate ceremony, and my theme was "Faith, Hope and Love." At the next day's commencement I sat between Principal Byron Saffell and Superintendent B.F. Stanton. A front page story in Red + Blue showed pictures of Dwight and Jean Neal, voted Outstanding Boy + Girl. How about them chickens?

Some other girls in our Homeworth, Ohio primary school class were Martha Rilmer and June Stewart Wagner. June's father brought the family from Latrobe, PA (home of the golfer Arnold Palmer). He also opened the first saloon/bar in the community. And, despite my father's warning, guess what? The town didn't immediately go straight to hell.

War

As I mentioned, at my high school graduation I was obliged to sit on the stage with Principal Byron Soffell and Superintendent B.F. Stanton. Since I had dated the principal's daughter, Ginny, I was even more nervous than usual. My oral response ended with, "And now abideth these three, Faith, Hope and Charity…Love."

That was June of 1942. Yes, America's naval base at Pearl Harbor had been bombed the previous winter. On the day after Pearl Harbor had been bombed, December 8, 1941 (a day after a day that will live in infamy), we all gathered in the AHS auditorium to hear President Roosevelt say, "Yesterday, our naval forces at Pearl Harbor were viciously and surprisingly attacked by the country of Japan." I had heard about the attack on Sunday, the 7th, on the radio, coming home from Messiah practice (the play, I wasn't rehearsing to BE Jesus).

I chose to stay on the farm from June of '42 until November of '43. Honestly, I could have stayed on the farm for the entire war, but instead I performed a rather deceptive act of patriotism. I wrote to my draft board in Lisbon, the county seat, and told them I was no longer needed on the farm with my dad, since he was farming with a neighbor, which was patently untrue. I never confessed to my father what I had done. I might observe here that, by that time, our family had already contributed two boys to the Service: Wilson and Paul. Brother Wilson was already in the 99th Division Band. Brother Paul had been deployed to the South Pacific in the Air Force. I would make three, three stars for Palmer and Doris, three stars in the window.

    I was called up in late November 1943, and Sister Ruth drove me to Salem (12 miles) to catch a train to Columbus, the Induction Station. Then I was stuck in Columbus for 2 or 3 days, awaiting assignment. While waiting, I met a local soldier, Verne Wooten, who invited me to his place for a meal. There I met his wife, Shirley, who tutored PhD students for their language requirement. More on that later.

    I took a train across the country, to Fort Lawton, in Seattle, Washington. I'll never forget getting up in the morning when we got to Idaho, and seeing that glistening sun-drenched jewel of a metropolis, Boise, Idaho.

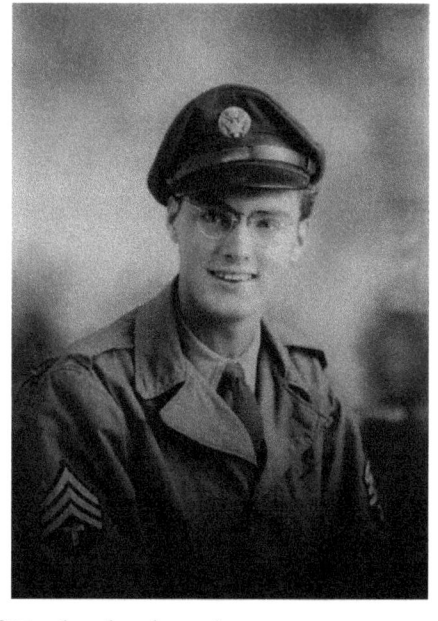

    Fort Lawton was a Port of Embarkation, but not my embarkation. I hadn't even been through Basic Training yet. No problem! Three weeks of Basic Training lay before me. In those twenty-one days, I honed my shooting skills on the rifle range, which, honestly were already pretty good. You put up a target and I'll of course hit it, to this day. I also crawled under wire on the training course, learning in the process the true and literal meaning of the phrase "Keep your butt down."

    One extra-curricular activity I remember is attending a USO dance and dancing with a girl who begins an evening, seeking adventure. Good dancer, good conversationalist, good evening. Oh, I found a fancy dance decoration for my dear mother, and sent it to her.

Soon I was sent clear across the country to my POE (point of embarkation), to be put on a troop ship bound for Europe. I took a transcontinental train trip, which landed me in New York, at what turned out to be my (POE) Port of Embarkation to the European Theater. New York City was my last glimpse of the USA until my time in this war that almost swallowed the Earth whole was finally done.

On the angry North Atlantic, our troop ship was crowded. We meticulously traversed the stormy, angry, bitterly cold sea. The Atlantic's twenty-foot waves produced beaucoup sea-sickness. Somehow I escaped the "heaves," at the same time as poor, short Eshelman, our "Mr. Five-by-Five," was feeding his breakfast to the fishes.

For some reason I made my way to the radio control room where the onboard (Disc Jockey) DJ Mac Bitter was spinning records. He welcomed me, asking me if I had anything I could do. And I said, "All I know is THIS IS WORTH FIGHTING FOR." He replied, "The mic is yours."

Here are the words I said that day:

> I saw a peaceful old valley
> With a carpet of corn for a floor
> And I heard a voice within me whisper
> This is worth fighting for.
> I saw a little old cabin
> And the river that ran by the door
> And I head a voice within me whisper
> This is worth fighting for.
> Didn't I build that cabin?
> Didn't I plant that corn?
> Didn't my folks before me

> Fight for this country?
> I gather my loved ones around me,
> And I gaze at each face I adore
> And I hear a voice within me THUNDER
> THIS IS WORTH FIGHTING FOR!

We eventually landed in Liverpool, England, and boarded buses to take us to our first overseas billet, where we were bivouacked in tents. Along the way, war-ravaged British children lined the side of the road, begging us for food and hope. Luckily we all had both of those in abundance. American GIs' generosity led to a lot of candy bars being tossed out the windows in their direction that day.

It was bitterly cold and wet, and I think I wet the bed the first night on foreign soil. Ouch! Shades of growing up with enuresis. I had to face it. I was a bed wetter. At home I slept on a straw tick. Back on the farm, if my "bed" was wet the next morning, we would just replace the straw. No chance of that here. I sent my bedding to the laundry. That chill struck me to the bone the first night, and that humiliation passed.

During WWII I was assigned to The Transportation Corps, and was stationed in Plymouth, England for several months, sent to live in private quarters — at the Barnecuts' house, in a tiny town in Cornwall called Dobwalls. Archie was 51 and his wife Margaret 49. They had been married for two years. Arch was unattractive, with big ears, a big nose, and big hands — but also with a similarly big heart. I would be loading ammunition at 1 AM and coming back (three blocks) to my room at the Barnecuts', I would always take off my shoes so I could steal silently past the Archie and Margaret's bedroom. I never got more than two steps past their bedroom when Mrs. B, in a loud stage whisper, would call out, "That you, Dee?!"

A week or so later the Barnecuts' niece came to visit — an attractive girl in her early twenties. Yes, she slept in the guest room, and of course, I had to tell her a bedtime story! (Disclaimer: Back in the states, I had made a proclamation to myself that I would return home a virgin. I made true on that pledge, barely…by the skin of my teeth. There were some mighty close shaves. It was a tense time, when no one really knew what tomorrow would bring. I was young, curious, and surrounded by so many desperate, war-tossed women. Needless to say, it wasn't the ideal recipe for continued virginity, but to carry the metaphor well past where it should have stopped, I, Dwight Freshley, am a determined chef.)

Soon after, the Station Master's lovely daughter came home for a two-week visit. Her name was Anne Palmer, and she was around 25-30 years old, attractive and attracted to me. She invited me to go on a picnic. "Bring your raincoat," she instructed, though it was a clear day. I thought that we would use our raincoats to put the food on, but no, she had a tablecloth for that. Tea time was interrupted by a love tryst. Again, like I said, I kept my chastity pledge, but dear Lord those British girls didn't make it easy.

In preparation for D-Day, in March and April, there were practice invasions by the 29th Division. After the second practice, I overheard guys of the 29th letting loose with the most creative profanity I'd ever heard. The practice exercises carried out that spring, "Duck 1" and "Duck 2," were being honed and exacted for the real thing.

When D-Day did come, I was guiding the 29th "Dough Boys" down to the "Hards" on to the LCIs (Landing Craft Infantry). Practice was done. Now, it was time for the test. Thus began the biggest military operation in history. 29th Division: You got your wish, and dozens of your division didn't make it back.

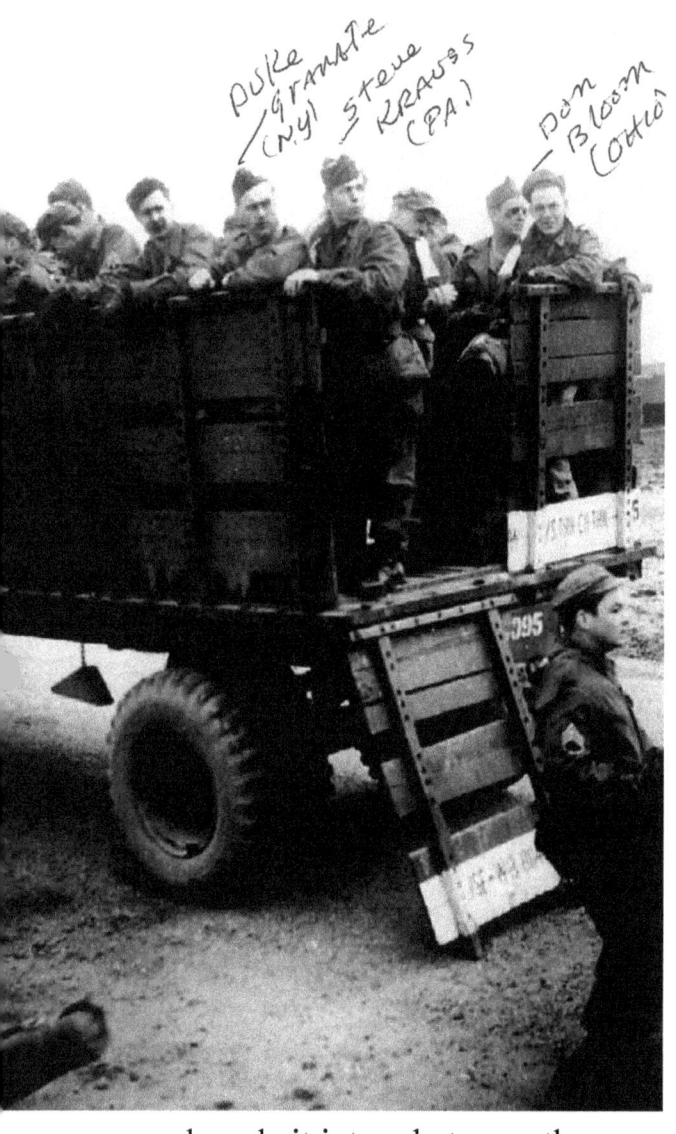

These guys wanted the real thing. Of course, when the 29th Division did lead the charge on D-Day (June 6, 1944), they lost 20% of their division in an extremely short amount of time. On that fateful day, I guided the troops to the "Hards" where the idling LCIs awaited. I vividly recall that the 29th following the same path they had in their practice invasions. Some of them told me later that, after they landed at Normandy and made it into what was, then, enemy territory, they had to keep their guards up every moment of every day. Even in darkest night in their makeshift camps, the latrines were ten or so yards away, and so the soldiers were cautioned not to disturb any of the foliage, because German Intelligence could detect changes on the ground.

In retrospect, I am awed at the magnitude of planning that went into this unparalleled operation undertaken by the Allies. They masterminded the largest military operation in history and, considering the peril of the recent past, the German beating taken by the determined but relatively small island of Britain, and (looking back now) the outcome, they won an impressive victory while playing an uncertain hand.

To be even just a small part of history as it was being made was exhilarating. But there was no time to blow one's own horn. Ammunition had to be delivered for Browning Automatic Rifles and submachine guns. Little did I know that I was even arming soldiers who came from close to my hometown: Bill Willard and Fred Shaeffer from Homeworth, Ohio, both of whom would pay the supreme price for their participation in D-Day. Bill was killed outright and Fred was listed as MIA — Missing in Action. That was a blow to the stomach. A year before, Fred and I had driven 40 miles West on Route 30 to visits Fred's girlfriend, "T," who recruited a girl for me, Sarah Moumaw (an undertaker's daughter — the potential for a smart remark here is almost limitless). There would be no follow-up to that date, although I think she may have written me a letter while I was in the Service.

The operation of the actual invasion, officially named Operation Overlord, conceived by President Franklin D. Roosevelt, Prime Minister Winston Churchill, and France's Charles De-Gaulle, and led by General Dwight D. Eisenhower, to effect the largest coalition of armed forces ever assembled in the free world, in order to oppose the most despicable and evil enemy of fascism, Adolph Hitler and his Italian henchman, Benito Mussolini, was a massive thing. Amazingly, the secret plans didn't leak to the Germans, despite their spy skills.

In the days following D-Day, I stayed at the English dockside, supervising the loading of ammunition — an operation executed in the middle of the night. Not long after, I was transferred to a Smoke Bomb Depot. My next job was sending smoke bombs to the European mainland for use in covering the Allied crossing of the Rhine.

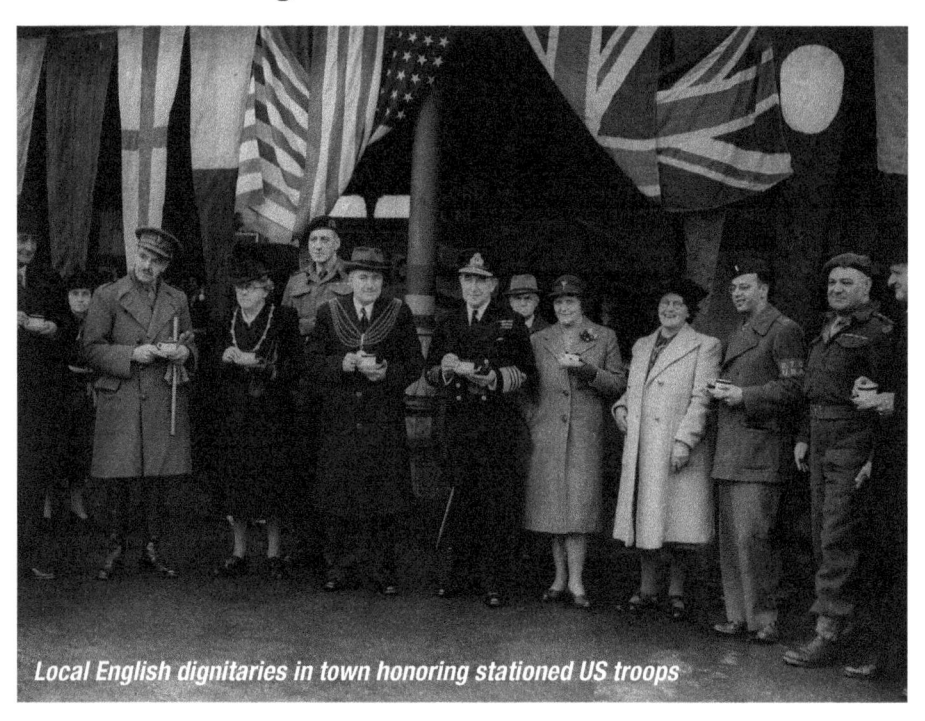

Local English dignitaries in town honoring stationed US troops

Fast Forward to the Serendipity Incident. A few months ago (from now), we had a panel of elderly veterans, speakers sharing their WWII experiences. One speaker was Hal Cooper, owner of Cofer's Lawn and Seed Company. Another was named Phil. Phil told us about his crossing the Rhine under a pillar of smoke. I suddenly realized that I was the one who sent the smoke bombs to cover Phil's crossing. Remarkable serendipity. Phil was fond of telling people that I was the first person he had met in Athens and this was before we realized our wartime connection.

I was later briefly assigned to the District Headquarters in Exeter. With that came a well-endowed maiden, whose memorable question still elicits cozy feelings in me. She pointed to her cleavage and asked, "Would you like to put your hand on my breast?" In a word, yes. Yes I would.

After D-Day and then Exeter, I was assigned to the Plymouth Road Railroad Station, where I became an R.T.O., and had an Army band to promote. When troops came though Plymouth, on transfer assignment or on leave (Furlough) they had to check in with us. The Army was pretty proficient at discovering our talents and using them to make the experience as pleasant as possible, given the situation.

The bane of my existence during the war was not a Nazi. It was an Allied soldier. It was an Allied soldier of a higher rank than I. It was an Allied soldier of a higher rank, my commanding officer, Captain Simpson. I hated that guy.

Simpson Mania. Item #1 I was pulling guard duty at Dormie House. It was late at night when Capt. Simpson drove up in his jeep. I did the standard military "Who goes there?" routine. Simpson acknowledged the general orders and started to drive off, but then suddenly stopped, backed the jeep up and threatened, "If you ever stop me again, I'll kill you, you son-of-a-bitch." I replied, "Captain, you need to go and sleep it off."

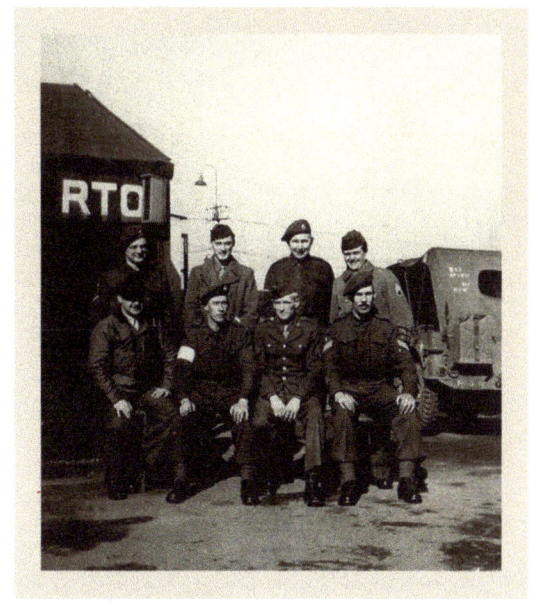

41

A second example of Captain Simpson's despicable behavior occurred when we were processing frostbite cases in a hospital about ten miles from Plymouth, in a little town called Tavistock. Simpson ordered a couple of us to coordinate the reception of these medical cases. We drove there a day early, as Captain Simpson recruited three nurses to "entertain" we three GIs. Yes, I passed up another (How can I say this delicately?) female "bonding" opportunity and enjoyed an hour in conversation with the girl, drafted against her will by my mortal enemy/commanding officer, Captain Simpson. Not only was he an angry guy and an Authoritarian bas#a*@, but he decided to round out his resume with the addition of Amateur Pimp as well.

Other, much less objectionable, personnel at North Road included Lenny Wiora from Chicago, Glenn Lanzig from Indiana Brighton, "Teddy Bear" Sgt. Baskwill (37-years-old and over 200 pounds), and Johnny Verloni from New York City. American regional differences dwindled in the 1940's, as we realized we were all in the same boat, metaphorically and sometimes literally.

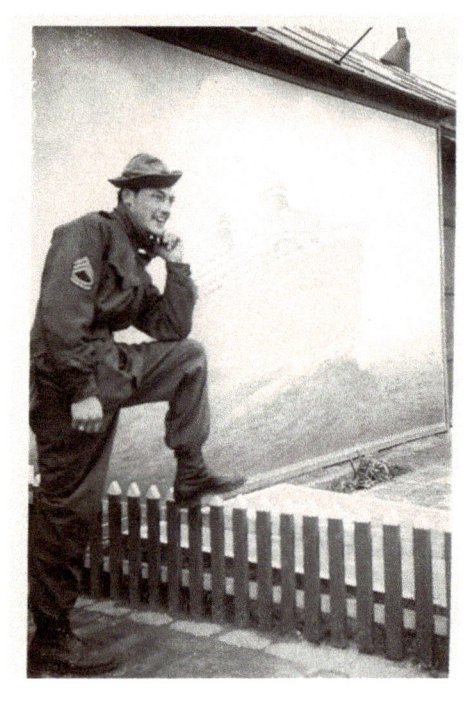

Soldiers were moved around a lot in World War II. For a while I was the only American rooming and boarding at Mrs. Andrews' boarding house in Plymouth. Mrs. Andrews had two children: Colin, in his 20's and in the British Army, and Olive, better known as "Ginger" because of her red hair. Ginger had a 9-month-old baby named Barry John, a beautiful child. Ginger was certain that the father, a Canadian sailor, would return and claim paternity. "Don't hold your breath, Ginger," because that didn't happen. Ginger would often come into my room, sit on my bed and tell me her troubles. She later determined that her only relief would come from committing suicide, but Ginger's first steps down that lonely road came in the form of running away from home a few times.

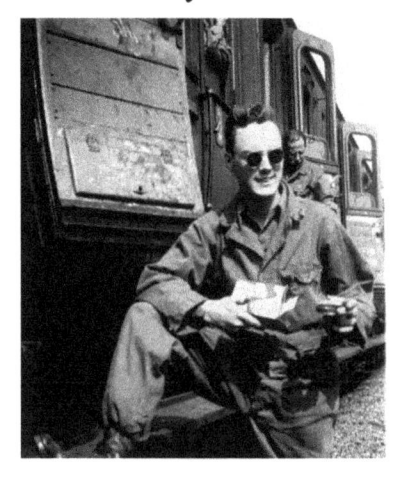

She cried "Wolf" a couple of times, abruptly leaving home and leaving worried family members and military boarders alike in her wake, all determined to chase her down. The second time Ginger ran away, there were three of us staying there at the boarding house on Crescent Drive. The two British soldiers headed for town to find her, and I went three blocks uphill to The Hoe — a five-foot boardwalk encircling the bay. Yes, it was from that very bay in 1620 that the Pilgrims sailed to America. How wonderful?

I finally encountered a British soldier — wearing a great coat (the British equivalent of the heavy American overcoat), and no hat. I addressed him politely, "Have you seen a young lady walking along here alone?" He replied in a cockney accent, "No, I haven't."

He and I walked together a few yards, down some steps and to a bench providing a lovely view of the bay. That night there was a ship standing out in the black, with lights emitting signals across the bay. After watching for five minutes or so, the lights climbed the steps on the other side and reached ground level. There was an iron railing protecting people from falling onto the rocks below. I paused, put my hand on the railing, and POW, that cockney chap clobbered me across the left ear, knocking me down, hurling my overseas cap and my G.I. glasses to the rocks below. I remember yelling, "You broke my glasses," and I was lost without my spectacles' correction of my nearsightedness. There was no apparent reason for the man's sudden attack, an attack which left me with a lifelong case of Tinnitus, but I later learned the extent of English resentment for we Americans. The Brits had "held down the fort" for the Allies, while Germany was gobbling up Europe one country at a time, France was being overrun by Nazis, and America was still making up its mind as to whether or not we wanted anything whatsoever to do with the war, beyond sending supplies. England had been bombed, bruised, beaten, and battered, but they held fast. Churchill's throaty voice echoed their resolve. "We will never surrender." And then, after Pearl Harbor, when America did enter the war, we turned the tide. The Brits were relieved to have a powerful ally, but that doesn't mean that they didn't feel some stereotypically English passive-aggression towards us. They used to mockingly say, "The Yanks are overpaid, oversexed and over here."

Back at Mrs. Matthews's place, my room was a made-over parlor, with a fireplace. As I said, it was not unusual for Ginger to slip in bed with me. I was her confidante and only friend. As difficult as it might be to believe, the Act was never consummated. The same went for lying down in front of the fireplace. I had pledged to come home a virgin, and I was adamant and farm-stubborn. An almost-duplicate event occurred on a sunny afternoon while on a picnic in a grassy patch across the river in Cornwall. Devonshire had Plymouth as its capital. After enjoying a prepared picnic, it was time for affectionate dessert. We initiated what we called in the states "an old-fashioned necking session." I'm afraid we worked ourselves up into a bit of a frenzy. I called a halt to it and sat back down. After cooling off, Ginger yelled at me. "If you ever get me worked up again without going all the way, I'll kill you, you son-of-a-bitch!" Sounding far too much like Captain Simpson for my taste, I discovered that Ginger had some issues. My virginity pledge probably didn't help.

The Dance. Plymouth had a hotel called The Continental, which regularly hosted dances. Loving to dance, it was just a matter of time before I would find The Continental. When I did, the first night I found myself on the sidelines, watching

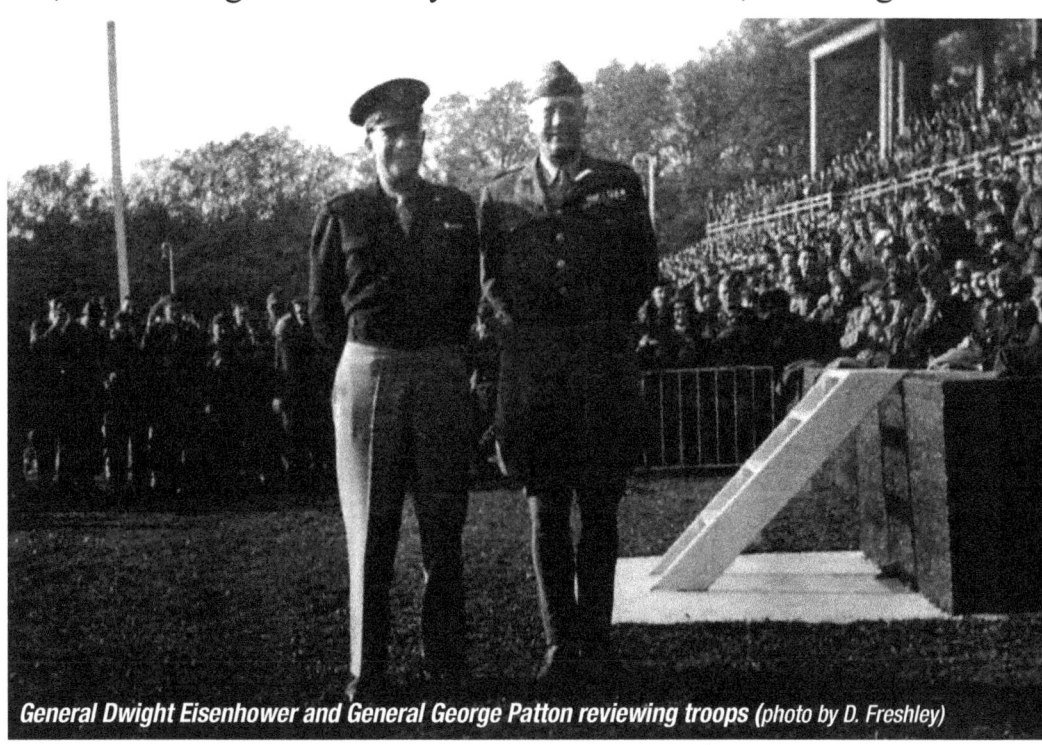

General Dwight Eisenhower and General George Patton reviewing troops (photo by D. Freshley)

the courting, the Jitterbugging and the soft, smiling sensations dancing by. I cut in to claim the next dance with an intoxicating beauty named Betty. And I broke another rule of mine by blithely not noticing the adornment on the third finger on her left hand. The huge diamond she wore should have told me that Betty was engaged, but I was far too struck by her beauty and joie de vive to notice. Betty covered my embarrassment, exclaiming, "I can read the sign on the next building!"

Later Betty caused my embarrassment by inviting me to tea on Sunday, the next day. I made my way from Cornwall to Devon and found a bus that would land me close to Mount Gold Avenue, where Betty lived. I do remember that not two blocks from the Plumb House there was a crater from a German Buzz Bomb. Too close for comfort. Along with Coventry and London, Plymouth was one of the hardest-hit targets of the German bombardment in England.

I guess it was on that visit that I played tennis with Mrs. Plumb (Anne). After playing a game that afternoon, we sat down to take off our shoes. It was a hot day and our feet had swelled, making it difficult to change shoes. I recall sitting on the ground, looking at our huge, swollen, sweating feet and roaring with laughter.

Soon I was transferred to Exeter County, next to Devon, to the District Office. There was always one female who came to visit. I don't remember her name, but I do recall that her breast size was 42. (Please do give me a break, dear readers. Keep in mind that I was young, naïve, inexperienced and thrust into something impossible to prepare for.) I think it was in Exeter that I met a soldier named, I swear to God, Sgt. Sherlock Holmes…and he wasn't even a Brit. He was from Washington State.

Later, I was transferred back to Plymouth, where I met Pat Locke, a vivacious strawberry blonde, back at my favorite dance hall home away from home, The Continental Hotel. I have never danced with another girl who, like Pat, seemed to not have a single bone in her back. Dancing with Pat Locke was like dancing with a fish, in a good way. I never met Pat's family, but we did take a bus trip together, to Torquay, England's equivalent of Miami Beach on a memorable occasion which was, unbeknownst to us, right around the corner.

May 8, 1945 finally arrived. I may not have known it on that day, but the war in Europe had finally ended. It was V-E Day. I celebrated with Pat Locke and hundreds of others. We took a classic British double-decker bus to Torquay, a beach resort full of excitement at the end of a long and nearly world-shattering war. What a glorious day. Pat swam in the bay and looked great in a bathing suit.

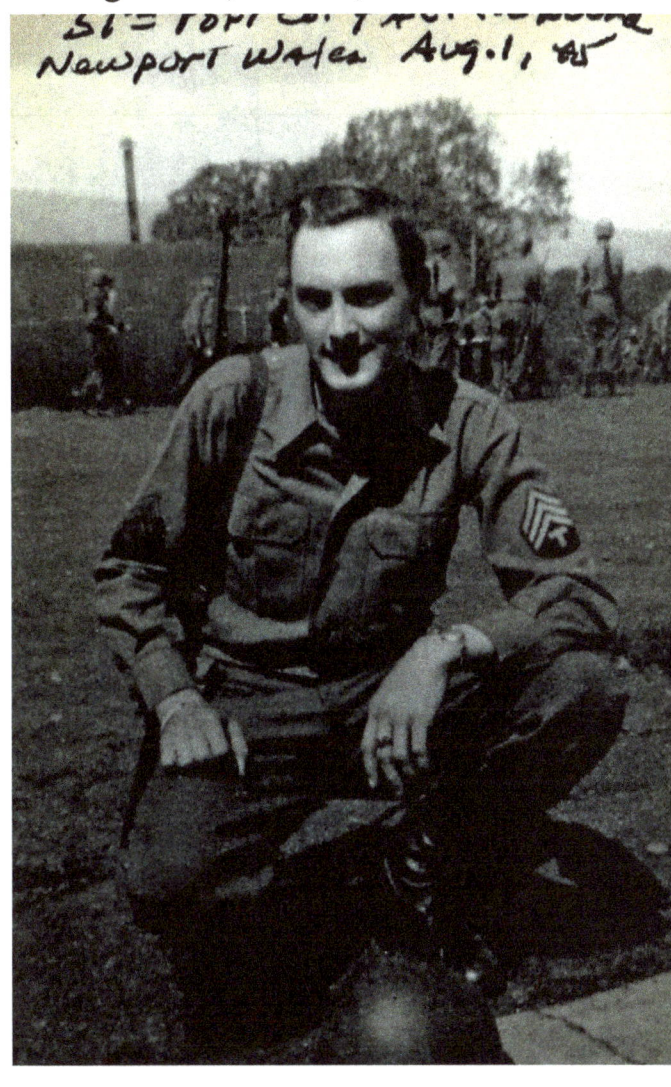

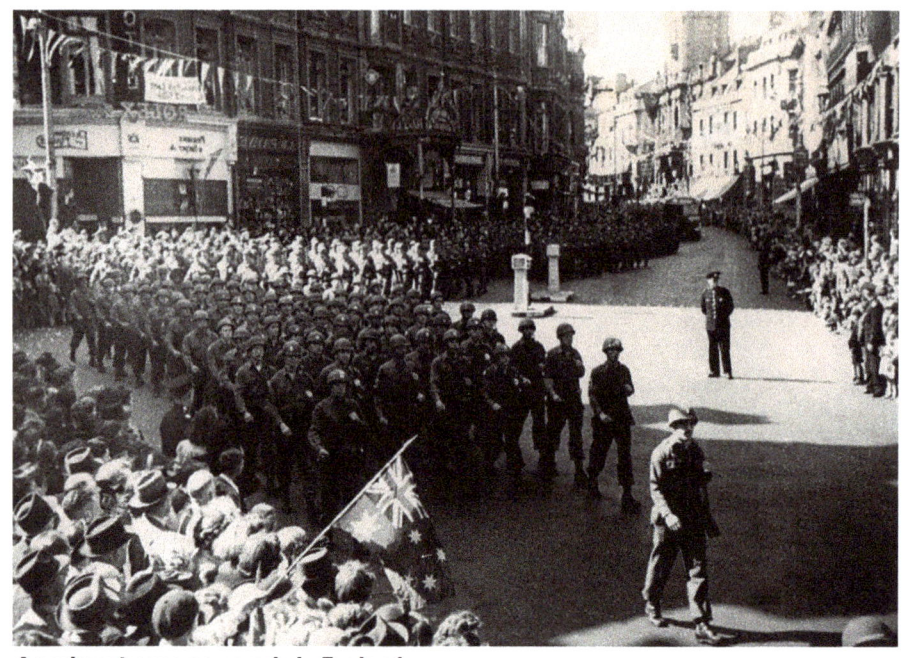

American troops on parade in England

America did, however, still have Japan to defeat. I was sent to Wales to prepare to be sent to the Far East. I was #90 on the ship's manifest. Then President Harry Truman calmly made a decision which would change the course of History, for he had in his hand the secret weapon with unimaginable power — The Atomic Bomb — the possession of which forever changed the course of the history of the world. The plane delivering this lethal weapon was the Enola Gay, piloted by James A. Doolittle. Goodbye Hiroshima and Nagasaki.

And where was Sergeant Freshley? In Wales, waiting for the other shoe to drop. And drop it did, albeit positively, with the arrival of V-J Day that very August. Visiting Margaret Williams and watching the Victory Parade in Newport, Wales are fond memories from those days. Margaret and I had no torrid romance, rather a satisfactory friendship.

During the war, I had never had a true furlough in the Army, so I decided I would dance in at least four venues:

1) Glasgow, Scotland
2) Edinburgh
3) Worcester &
4) London

In Glasgow, I met Mamie McCaffey at an Amateur Dance Competition, and we danced the night away. When we finally tired and went outside, it was almost as bright as daylight. "I try to forget/The day that we met/But raindrops keep beating your name." Mamie went down her lane with a goodnight kiss and I started back to my Army digs. I remember it like it was yesterday, thinking that morning, "It's so bright out here that I could read a newspaper."

I never got to see him perform, but Bob Hope was the big USO attraction, the main event wherever he stopped off to cheer up weary troops. He would come on stage with two Red Cross civilian women, dispensing coffee and doughnuts to the crowd. Everyone loved his shows. I almost met him, coming within 20 feet, but then got lost in the crowd.

When I looked for a place to stay I was directed to a lady with a room to rent. She showed me to the room and then asked, "What time would you like me to knock you up in the morning?" ("America and England, two countries separated by a common language." I'm pretty sure that's an Oscar Wilde line.) My follow-up line, attempting to clear things up, was, "I beg your pardon?"

The port of Glasgow was the embarkation point for returning U.S. soldiers (but not yet me) and their "first class" accommodations were on the Queen Mary and the Queen Elizabeth. I was given the passenger list (called the "manifest") to admit people onboard with.

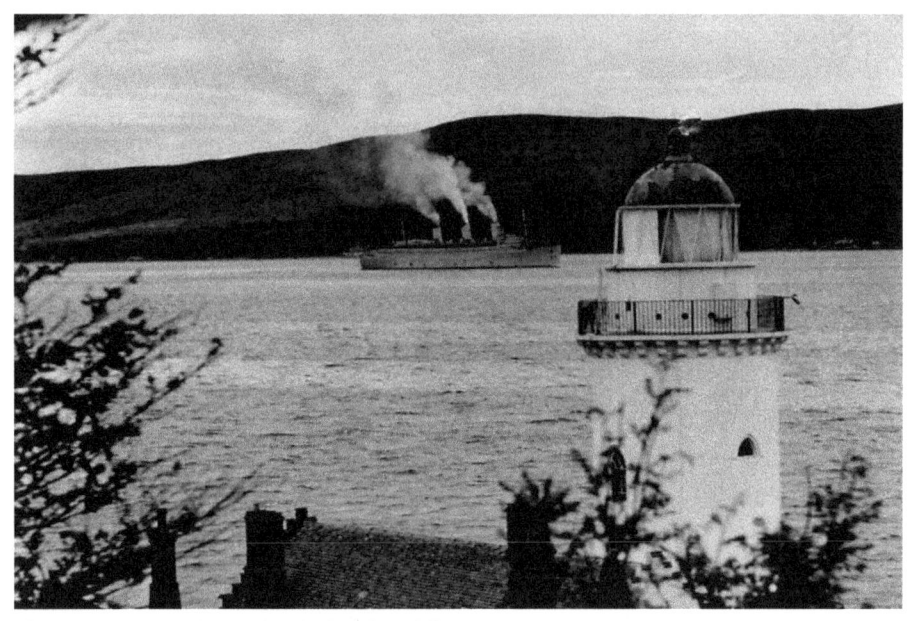

Queen Mary coming in loaded with soldiers

With V-J Day (Hooray), the biggest war in history had ended! I was sent to Paris and billeted on the Champ d'Elysie. On the streets of gay Paree I learned what "Zig, Zag, Baby" meant, but again I somehow managed to keep my virginity in tact. (Hey, it's not what you think. I'm complaining, not bragging.) One enduring memory of those days was the amazing fact that I could step out of my Parisian billet, turn right and a mere hundred yards away was the Arc de Triumph. Alas, the action scene of my war story ended and I was to be sent to Frankfurt, Germany, to be housed in the Furstenberger Schule (school), until the end of my tour of duty. I'll just share one more thing about the war, not about my experience, rather my brother's. My brother Wilson had joined the Army before I did, and was put in the 99th Division Band. During the Battle of the Bulge the band was pressed into medical units. The 99th Division stormed through Europe, liberating towns, and, in the process, liberating souvenirs from German houses. Wilson took a little rose-like flower encased in glass. Forty-five years later, Wilson went back to Germany, found the house and put the flower in glass back on the wall of its former home.

When we were both in Germany after the war ended, I got a weekend pass to visit Wilson, taking a train from Frankfurt. Wagner's home was just twenty miles north. I hitched a ride on the cab of a semi trailer which was deadheading. With the biting cold and my arms around the warm exhaust pipe it was windy and was one hell of a ride. I don't remember much about the renowned composer's birthplace.

I also reunited with Wilson in Paris. I have a great photo of us both in front of La Sacre Coeur.

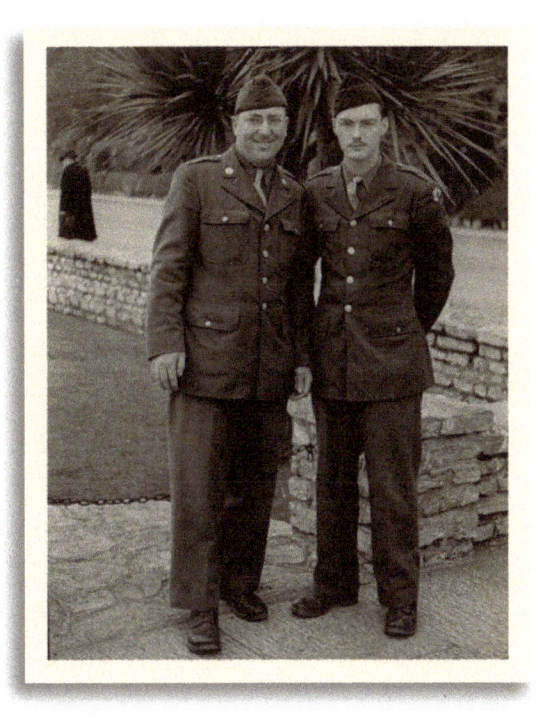

The War shaped my life, as it did with so many of us, but when it was over, it was over, and time for me to return home and begin my "real life." I still had no idea what my real life would be like, but nonetheless I was anxious to get started on it.

51

College

Something they never tell you in the recruitment offices is how slow military time passes once the fighting is over. It was time for me to leave the ETO (European Theater of Operations). The war was over in both theaters, and we were all anxious to get home. But military time is slow. While waiting, I decided to do something productive with my time, participating in a Social Science survey I partially invented. I devised a test of 30 questions, all with five alternative answers, administered in order to compile personality statistics for the Army. The test measured, among other things, personality types: from Authoritarian to Authoritative to Cooperative/Democratic. I filled out a very long questionnaire and asked other GIs (and civilians if they spoke decent English), to do the same. Though I didn't know it at the time, this would be a foreshadowing of the social science degree in Speech Communications I would later earn at The Ohio State University, taught by Dr. Franklin H. Knower. (He would often fall asleep while lecturing, but otherwise, he was a good teacher.)

In Frankfurt, Germany I met Irmgart, a waitress in the dining hall. She invited me to join her family for a meal in their home. I'd never been in a real German home before, and was kind of excited. I remember being full and politely declining to take dessert. The next day Irmgart told me that her mother thought I'd refused the dessert because I thought she was trying to poison me. Of course, I hadn't thought that. Why would I? The war was over. And, if I had thought they were trying to poison me, why would I assume they'd only poison the dessert? The day we were loaded in trucks and headed for the POE (Port of Embarkation), a German band serenaded us with a brass version of "Sentimental Journey"! "Gonna take a sentimental journey..." I don't think the Germans realized the irony.

I came home on a troop ship in April 1946, mustered out of Camp Atterbery, Indiana, and took a bus to Canton, Ohio, where someone picked me up. The reunion with Mother was poignant and joyful. She had been my most faithful correspondent for 2&1/2 years. I never received a single letter from Dad.

Boarding a train at Canton, I found a compartment. Later, when I needed to use the restroom, I went down the corridor to the Men's Room. There was a black soldier in there, looking at himself in the mirror, fingers curled at the bottom of his sideburns, saying aloud, "Oh, I'd give anything to change this black skin to white." He never saw me, but he left an impression. (Who could blame him for thinking that at the time?) My views on race relations would never be the same.

I was anxious to begin college and wanted to follow in my brothers' footsteps, attending North Central College in Naperville, Illinois, from which Wendell and Paul had graduated in 1941.

I enrolled at North Central College for the fall semester. During that summer, I stayed with my brother, Wendell, in Perrysburg, Ohio in the NW sector of the Buckeye State. Wendell was married to Virginia Farley. They had two children: Dorcas and Mark. Sadly, Virginia died of Bulbar polio just one year short of the invention of the Salk Polio Vaccine. Wendell then married a woman named Ruth and she had a premature pregnancy, having to remove the baby after only six months of gestation, leaving the child blind and mentally-retarded. But the child lived. Facially, Wendy's child, Joylene, resembled our sister Ruth.

Though she could not manage Braille, Joylene had some amazing vocal talent. She could sing, "Summertime" and you would swear it was Marian Anderson, the popular African-American songstress who sang at The White House. Or Joylene could favor you with Barbara Streisand's "The Way we Were." I wish Barbara and Bob (Redford) could've heard Joylene sing.

When I finally arrived at North Central in the fall of 1946, I took a room in the home of Cora Frost, on Center Street, two blocks from Old Main. Early on I started dating Carolyn Steele, a buxom, dark-hued beauty from South Bend. Carolyn and I were serious. She was the first girl I'd ever gone steady with. Carolyn roomed in Bolton Hall and we regularly "got friendly" on the davenport in the parlor, so familiar that Housemother Miss Meyer once caught us in the act. I said goodnight to her at the door…frosting on the cake!

Carolyn and I were "an item" for two years. Unfortunately for me, the end was rather tragic and predictable. What came next might be properly called "The Blame Game." My dear brother Wendy (Wendell) is not here to defend himself, but I'll let this family secret slip anyway. Wendy discouraged me from continuing my relationship with Carolyn for this misperception/reason — When Carolyn would meet someone new, she'd scrunch her shoulders and flash her eyes coquettishly. I don't think it was conscious flirtation. She was just friendly and full of life. Quite possibly it was just the power of the male ego assuming certain intentions. It happens. Wendell thought she was "coming on" to him! I guess he figured that if she would come on to my preacher brother, she'd come on to anyone.

Wendell's "advice" led me to ask Carolyn if we might date other people for a couple of weeks. "Worst decision of my life." It seems she took her next move right out of some female coed playbook of the day, running in a straight line from me and into the arms of the quarterback of the football team, Johnny Lubbach. Carolyn never looked back, and I was left holding an empty dream.

My junior year at NCC was highlighted by a run for the Student Body President. I was running against Gordon St. Angelo, a "real" politician, who dated as many coeds as he could, merely for their votes. There was an important conference at Michigan State University which I attended, sponsored by The United Nations. I was supposed to give a campaign speech to the student body on a Friday afternoon. I decided it was more important for me to attend the UN gathering about Race Relations, where I met a wonderful girl I called Queen Esther, who cemented my position on the need for better race relations. Knowing I would not be on campus, I asked Bruce Reinhart to deliver my student body presidential hopeful speech. He was handsome and had a great voice. (I had dated Bruce's sister, Jean, a few times when she and I were freshmen, and later I truly did "go steady" with her --- and even later, I ended up marrying her.) I won the election, by the way.

Before reintroducing myself to Jean Reinhart, I had one of those experiences which became so indelibly imprinted on my brain that I couldn't forget it even if I were in a coma. On the first of October, 1949 I had a date with Rose Hodel, who was permitted to take "late leave," of (Gasp!)11:30. I remember our going to see the Freshman-Sophomore Tug of War and

I remember exactly where I parked the car on the grass, in an area students often used for "necking." We had been there only a few minutes when my driver's side door opened and a male voice said authoritatively, "This is a hold-up!" He stuck a gun in my ribs. Instinctively, I pushed the window with my left hand and socked him on the chin, knocking him back about ten feet. I leapt from the car and rushed him. He was still on the ground. Before I hit him again, he plaintively pleaded, "Gimme fifty cents, give me a dollar, and I won't do anything more to you." (Incidentally, this is not an effective robbery technique if employed at precisely the same time as your "victim" is atop you, pummeling you in the face.)

    I looked for something to hit the would-be robber with, but finding nothing, I called for Rose to go into the glove compartment and get me the bottle of tar remover inside. I yelled, "Hit him over the head!" As I held him down, she broke the bottle over his forehead, and Mister Ernest B. Knight (the attempted burglar's name) gagged as the fumes reached his eyes. I yelled to Rose to drive the car around while I "finished off" Mr. Knight. Rose returned to me, saying nervously, "I can't find the starter."

    "Never mind," I frantically replied, "Just get in the car." I hit Mr. Knight one more time, for good measure, and ran to the driver's seat. As we drove away from the clearing, we saw another car parked there. Concluding that it must've been the robber's, we memorized the license plate number as I pulled out onto Jefferson Avenue, a street that led right to the local police station, downtown, and right up the hill to the middle of the North Central College campus.

    I learned later that Ernest B. Knight was mentally-ill, and hid his violent compulsions from the world. He was a kind of Dr. Jekyll/Mr. Hyde character, a respected church elder by day, and a monster by night, abusing his family to such an extent that the police found some truly disturbing evidence, which I won't detail here, when they raided his home.

Being the Student Body President, and worried about the inevitable publicity after the foiled robbery attempt, I felt compelled to travel directly to the home of N.C.C. President C.R. Geiger, and dramatically tender my resignation. He lived veritably across the street. I went to his house, and Mr. Geiger invited me in. I told him my purpose for coming, after which he put his hand on my shoulder and said philosophically, "Dee, don't worry about the publicity. It will be gone in three or so weeks."

A reporter from the *Chicago Sun Times* came to campus to report on the incident. In fact, I described what had happened to two reporters, one was the memorable Ziggy Field of the Chicago Tribune, who had a car with a telephone in it, a rarity for the times. Ziggy finished the interview in the car, got out, walked around the car and took my picture with my arm resting on the window. This pose was in the next edition of the "Trib." While I was talking to another reporter, the phone rang, and it was Jack Koten, a prominent Junior who was there. He asked, "Dee, have you seen the Tribune yet?" It was 7-7:30 and the Trib was a morning paper. "Let me read the headline for you. CO-ED BEATS THRILL ROBBER." (Remember her breaking the bottle over his head?)

I suffered some humiliation, especially at home in Ohio when the postmaster's husband asked me during Christmas holidays, "Hey, Dwight, where were you during the hold up? Under your dash?"

However, I received a letter of warm support from Rose's father, Mr. Hodel, who thanked me for saving his daughter from being raped. I had driven down to Berkeley, West Virginia the previous summer, to visit the Hodel family, where I found out that Mr. Hodel owned two newspapers and a radio station...and I dearly wanted to go into radio at the time. Perhaps, had I taken a slightly different path, I could have had a career in radio, or even landed my then-dream job, on the ground floor of the budding new medium of television. That visit was warm and cordial. I remember thinking after the Chicago Tribune coverage of the story that my dating days at NCC were over, "No girl is going to feel safe going out with me!"

I believe I took the, now famous, coed Rose to the Junior-Senior Prom. Louis Bloede took Jean Reinhart — the future Mrs. Freshley. I had dated Jean a few times as a freshman, but it wasn't until three years later, as a senior, that we both felt something more intense than merely dating. As you can see from her pictures, Jean was a strikingly beautiful woman. What you can't necessarily see was how kind, diligent, generous and loving she was.

That spring semester, at a celebration of spring, the senior class honored the new life of the year with a trip to Indiana Dunes State Park. I still have the photo of my roommate Paul Stiffler jokingly pretending to wring Mary Jean Ultzman's neck! Good times.

A week or so later I played a game of softball and had a bad hip hit me in the face, breaking my glasses and cutting my left eye, compelling me to wear a bandage over that eye. I think Mother did the first-aid. For the next month or so, I looked like a suave Midwestern pirate, missing only a cutlass and a mustache...at least that's how it settled in my mind.

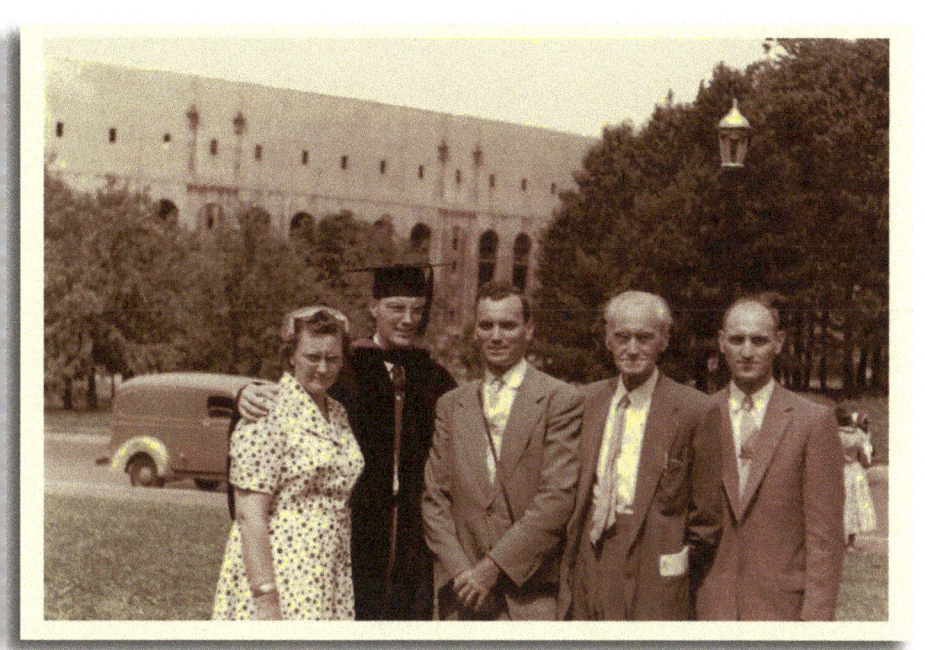

College graduation: (L-R) Sister Ruth, Dwight, Brother Paul, Father Palmer, Brother Wilson

Graduation Day finally arrived and guess who came to see me? My dear Mother. She had to travel a good 400 miles to see her baby boy finally graduate. It made my day.

Later that month I took Jean (still then Jean Reinhart, but not for long) to Ohio. CONFESSION TIME — On that trip Jean wore a yellowish-orange dress and no bra, which did make the trip vastly more interesting. I had a hard time keeping my eyes on the road. To cap off that memorable visit, I proposed marriage to Jean. She lived at home for the first three years of college, but had moved into the Craylor Hall dormitory for her senior year. Oh, she said "Yes" to my question, by the way. Thank God.

My major project in the summer of 1950 was the Midwestern tour of recruiting students for North Central with my friend Floyd Thompson. The previous year we had been Homecoming Co-Chairmen. Floyd and I both loved our alma mater and wanted to share that love with others. Let's face it, North Central was good to the Freshley family. With that spirit of pride and adventure, Floyd and I took off in June and headed for South Dakota, specifically The Black Hills, participating in all of the expected hi-jinks along the way. I remember at one point, on a road not heavily-traveled (of which there are plenty in sparse, rural South Dakota.), Floyd getting out and lying in the middle of the road, his big stunt of the trip. Looking back from the vantage point of today, the only truly memorable part of the trip occurred at the foot of The Black Hills. We met a bearded native, Ed Ryan, hawking his book about this famous landmark. Of course, we bought a copy and thoroughly enjoyed visiting with this colorful, bearded character. In addition, Floyd and I visited several summer camps in those three months, and served as enthusiastic representatives of our beloved college.

My home base at that time was in Southern Illinois. I was staying with Jean's folks. I commuted from Naperville to Evanston, to begin studying for my MA at a prestigious institution of higher learning. Northwestern had one of the best-known graduate programs in Speech Communication in the country. Memorably, I took three Oral Interpretation courses, "Oral Interpretation of Poetry" taught by the famous Charlotte Lee (who wrote the textbook), "Oral Interpretation of Drama" from Alvina Krause, and "Oral Interpretation of Prose" from Robert Breen, who had a keen aesthetic sensibility, once memorably abruptly stopping his lecture to bless out a tardy student.

    I stayed at Northwestern for that summer and experienced the happy serendipity of having my brother, Paul, get his MA on the exact same day as I got mine! I took a Speed Education course from the well-known Karl Robinson, who also wrote the textbook. Incidentally, at the time I was thinking at the time of becoming a Debate Coach, one of the worst ideas I've ever had, and we'll get to that a bit later. In retrospect, I might should've gone to the University of Wisconsin, which had a good program in radio & television. But, with a fiancé and future family to support I felt like I needed more security, and so, to quote the great Yankee catcher Yogi Berra, I came to a fork in the road…and I took it! It may have been the wrong fork, or maybe even the wrong road altogether, but I did enjoy teaching.

The next portion of my life was a hybrid experience of beginning to work in Academia while still being a recipient of the rewards of intellectual pursuit myself. I was working on a doctorate while dipping my toe into the pond of a teaching career which, along with my new family, would dominate the remainder of my life.

Career and Family

THE REST OF THE STORY

And now, for Jean Reinhart Freshley, my wife of 63 years, may I please request a salutation, a bow, a round of applause, a six-gun salute from you all. There are no appropriate words for this inimitable creature who kindly committed to be my wife. Jean Reinhart had grown up in West Naperville, two blocks from the local swimming pool, which she frequented. In her high school yearbook, in the picture of the girls' basketball team, Jean is sitting in the front row, center, holding the ball. That was before I knew her, but even a quick glance at that photo is enough to reassure me that I made the right choice with the biggest decision of my life.

Jean and I dated a few times my freshman year, and she had later dated Bob Blessman her freshman year, but was free in January of her senior year…and so was I. Later, after our honeymoon in September of 1950, Jean lived at home and walked ½ mile to classes. She really wanted to go to college and live on campus, but her parents simply couldn't afford to send her. I was the lucky recipient of their tight budget. I still pinch myself at my good fortune at meeting her. Jean was strikingly attractive, smart and athletic. We really didn't start "going steady" until my final semester of college. A major

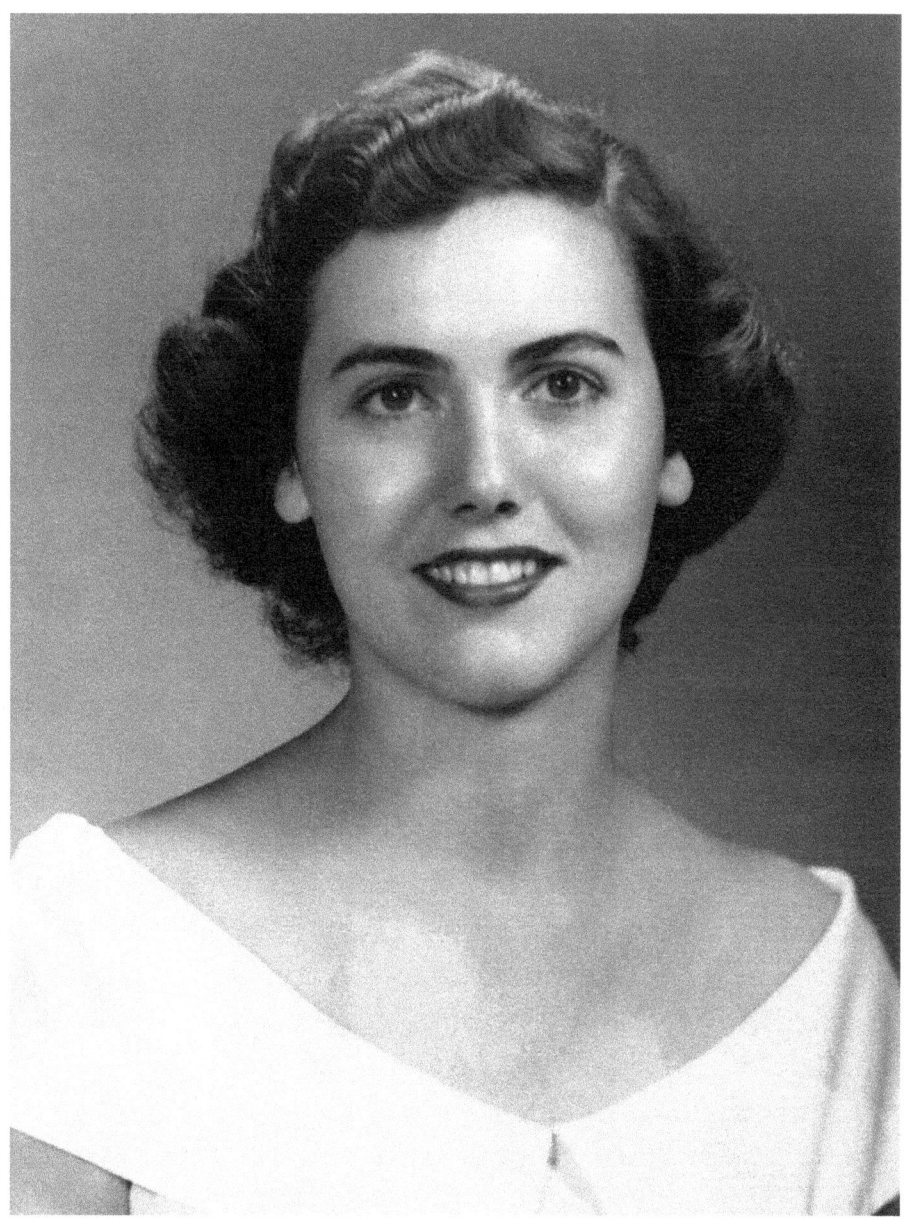

memory from the spring of 1950, now immortalized in a photograph which shows me coming out of the Reinharts' front door with a large patch over my right eye from a softball game, was the way Jean's family immediately embraced and welcomed me into their circle. Seeing my latest injury, Jean's mother, Freida, empathized. I was one lucky son-in-law to have in-laws like Freida and Chet. We'd drive into Naperville at 7 or 8 PM, where a delicious meal was always waiting. She was the best.

Chet, Jean's father, was incomparable. A builder, he built a hospital for our church mission in Nigeria, in a place called Joss. He also built eight buildings for the local women's college. When he was returning home in a British Jeep he brought along a missionary couple, who had probably never met a man like Chet, a man who would rise at 4 AM to capture the perfect lighting for a photograph of a flower opening up. Chet loved adventure, and would drive that Land Rover through town pretty fast. Woe to those who got in his way.

When he returned home from his African mission trip, Chet resumed his building career, erecting two duplexes across from his house. One day, while working on the roof, he fell off and broke his right leg, having to lay in bed and rest it in a sling suspended from the ceiling. When the nurse came to bathe him, he instructed her, "You wash as high as possible and as low as possible, and I'll wash the 'possible.'" That was my father-in-law in a nutshell. Funny, passionate, kind, generous and never having met a stranger. Jean had such amazing parents that she was destined from day one to be as exceptional as she did, of course, eventually become.

To help Chet that first summer I was courting his daughter, I tried to show off my farm skills, carrying wheelbarrows of "mud" (concrete). Trying to negotiate that heavy wheelbarrow up an eight-inch plank, and I weighing only 150 lbs., was no easy task. Somehow, with such strong motivation, I managed.

Jean and I had wedding invitations printed for December 10, 1950. That year I was teaching and finishing up my doctoral

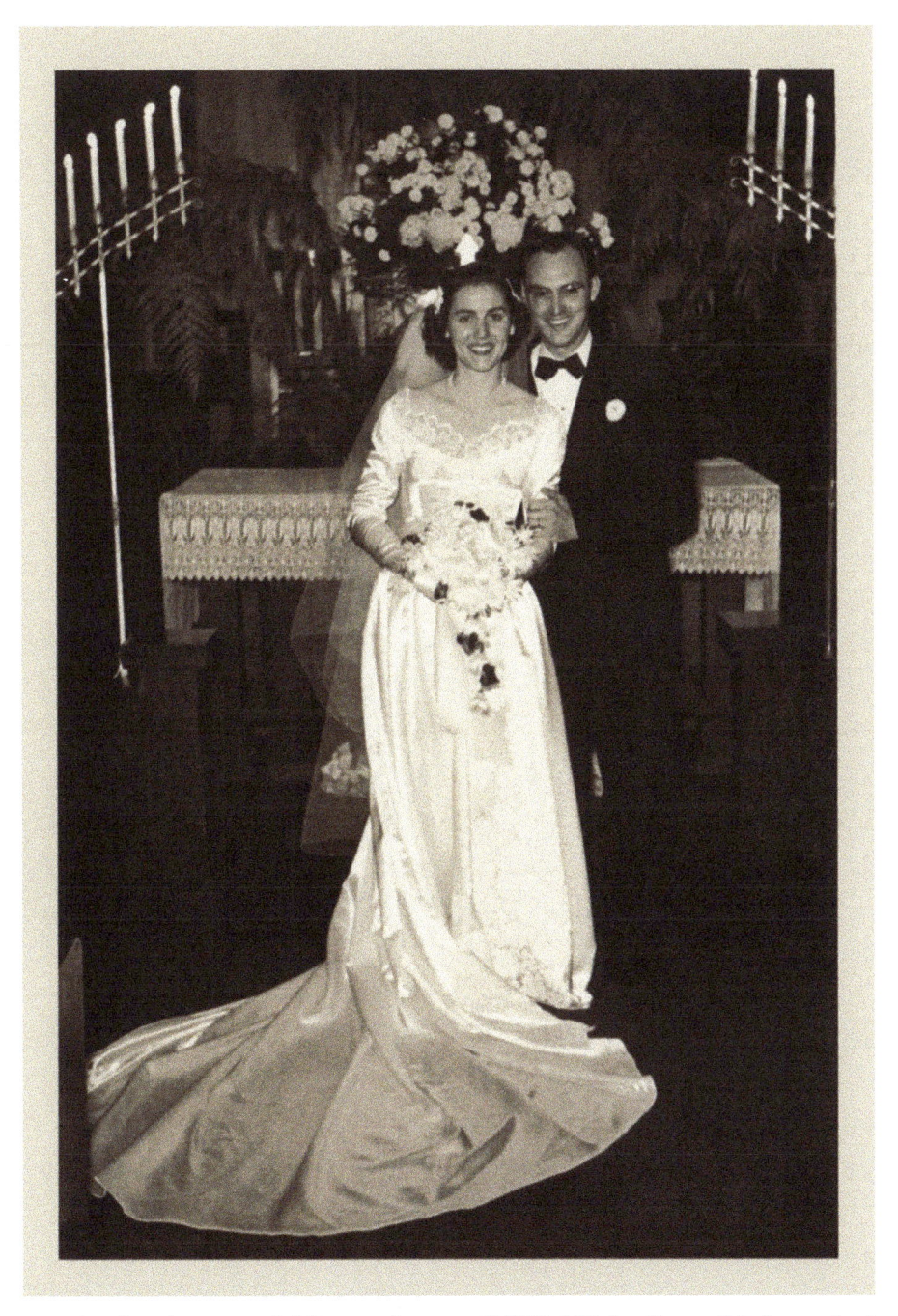

work. On August 24 I was in my OSU (Ohio State University) office, finishing grading exams, when the phone rang. It was my very pregnant wife. Our first child was due September first, but Phil had a mind of his own. We knew it would be a boy, and had chosen the name Philip Dwight, nicknamed "PhD." Since I was about to receive my doctorate on Thursday, August 26, the Columbus Dispatch picked up the story and put it on the bottom of the front page with the headline OSU STUDENT RECEIVES TWO PhD'S IN ONE WEEK. Needless to say, I preferred this to my previous newspaper headline.

After Phil's birth and the end of my PhD studies, I ended up accepting a position as a Debate Coach at Lehigh University in Bethlehem. In Karl Robinson's summer class, I researched the debate topics for the next year, on wages and price controls.

(Let me say now that I now realize that I wasn't ever cut out to be a Debate Coach, but I did it for years at two great schools: Lehigh and Vanderbilt University.)

Debaters at Lehigh included Bill Stafford, Paul Handwork and Elliot Barnet. I was a real novice at coaching debate. On reflection, my recipe for having a team was simple: start with very bright students, teach them the fundamentals and then point them to the library.

H. Barrett Davis was the Theatre Director and the Director of Fine Arts at Lehigh. He had a craggy face and a deep voice. Davis was a good boss. Despite my misgivings about coaching debate, I gained respect from my debaters as I "tooled" them around Brooklyn at the Brooklyn College Debate Tournament. Docile Dwight became a demonstrative, dangerous, devilish taxi driver.

It was in Brooklyn that I wrote two songs: "Wanted" and "Supersonic Santa Claus." The men's Chorus Director George Ganse added in the chords, so I could take them to New York to get published. I took my songs to Philadelphia to get a professional to "put them on wax," period industry slang for recording the songs. My contact turned out to be Candy Anderson, who had been on the popular Arthur Godfrey radio program. She cut the record, for $100, if I remember correctly. I took the demo to several music publishers. Everywhere it was the same answer — "We already have our own writer." Interestingly enough, that fall Perry Como came out with a hit song, also called "Wanted."

Orators Eye State Debate Tourney; Clement to Welcome 120 Speakers

By Gary Cohen

Speakers and debaters from twelve Tennessee colleges will vie for honors here Jan. 31 and Feb. 1 in the annual Tennessee Forensic Tournament. Governor of Tennessee Frank G. Clement and Chancellor Harvie Branscomb will welcome some 120 competitors in Neeley Hall, Friday the 31st.

Vanderbilt, in a host role for the first time, is defending the senior debate championship of this particular tournament won last year by Joe Sills and Chester Burns.

The weekend contest includes competition in: senior men's debate; junior men's debate; women's debate; extempore, impromptu, after dinner speaking, original oratory, and peace oratory. Winning speeches in the peace oratory contest will compete in national competition.

A Sweepstakes Award is awarded the school amassing the best record in the tournament. David Lipscomb College of Nashville is defending champion.

Visiting colleges will be: Belmont College and David Lipscomb of Nashville; University of Tennessee of Knoxville; Memphis State College; Middle Tennessee State College of Murfreesboro; Tennessee Polytechnical Institute of Cookville; Carson-Newman College; Lincoln Memorial University; and East Tennessee State College of Johnson City.

For Vanderbilt Burns and Sills; Fred Beesley and Vastine Stabler; and Stan Ruby and George Stern will compete in the senior men's debate. Junior men's debate entries are Joe Roby and Tom Templin; Barbee Lyon and Howard Orebaugh; and Marshall Wellborn and Clark Tidwell. Judy Lefkovits and Pat Haggard will enter the women's debate division.

Headquarters for the tournament will be Room 1 in Calhoun Hall. Students of Vanderbilt and near by high schools will serve as timekeepers.

Dr. Dwight Freshley and Mr. Ken Pauli of the fine arts department are the faculty co-ordinators of the tournament.

VU Debaters Excel In Millsaps Tourney

The Vanderbilt debate squad marked up a 12-12 score for the Millsaps College debate tournament held Jan. 10 and 11 at Jackson, Miss., with one varsity team going to the semi-finals. Joe Sills, a Nashville junior, highlighted Vandy's showing by winning the first place gold medal for extemporaneous speaking in a field of more than 50 contestants.

Vanderbilt's two varsity and two junior teams all remained in competition after the preliminary rounds held on Friday. To be eligible for the eliminations the next day, teams had to win two out of four debates; all four established 2-2 records.

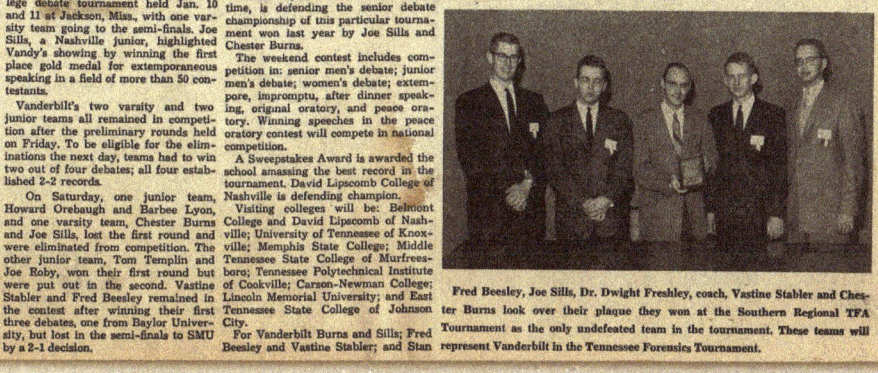

On Saturday, one junior team, Howard Orebaugh and Barbee Lyon, and one varsity team, Chester Burns and Joe Sills, lost the first round and were eliminated from competition. The other junior team, Tom Templin and Joe Roby, won their first round but were put out in the second. Vastine Stabler and Fred Beesley remained in the contest after winning their first three debates, one from Baylor University, but lost in the semi-finals to SMU by a 2-1 decision.

Fred Beesley, Joe Sills, Dr. Dwight Freshley, coach, Vastine Stabler and Chester Burns look over their plaque they won at the Southern Regional TFA Tournament as the only undefeated team in the tournament. These teams will represent Vanderbilt in the Tennessee Forensics Tournament.

Incidentally, there recently had been two gangsters in Pennsylvania who had help a couple hostage for several hours. It was a popular story of the day, on which both Perry and I, somewhat, based our songs. Como's song was quite popular, doubtlessly aided by the fact that he was Perry Como. The lyrics to my "Wanted" are in an Appendix at the back of the book.

Lehigh didn't take home a lot of medals in that Brooklyn tournament, but my debaters were effective, especially Bill Stafford and Paul Hardwood. Al Kappar, sometime debater,

67

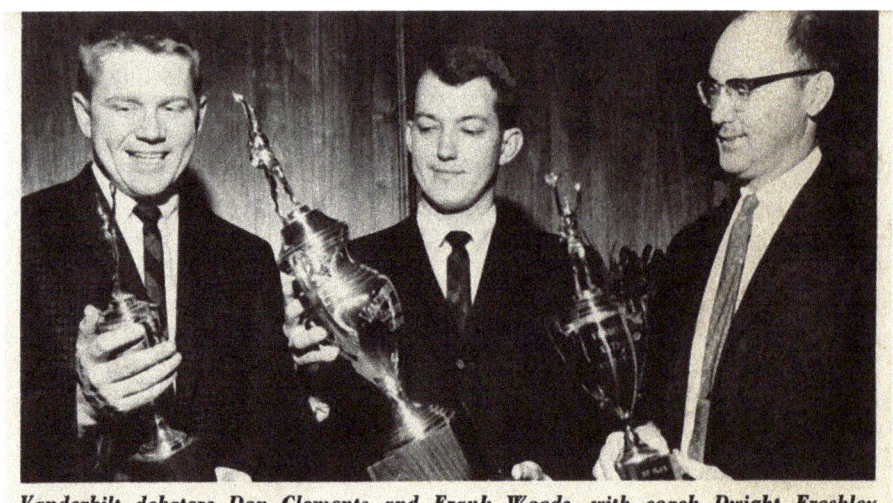

Vanderbilt debaters Don Clements and Frank Woods, with coach Dwight Freshley

big-time actor, and Elliott Barnett, a Jewish kid from New York, picked up valuable argumentative experience too.

A Lehigh English professor, Cloyd Criswell, and his lovely wife were good friends to Jean and me. Cloyd was also a painter and Jean and I bought one of his best works, a rail fence, which I related to, having grown up on a farm with similar fences. That painting now is displayed prominently in my son, Phil, and his wife, Marilee's, home in nearby Watkinsville, Georgia.

Accompanying the Criswells was the dramatic event of his having been mugged in downtown Philadelphia.

I became active in the DAPC (Debate Association of Pennsylvania Colleges) with new professional friends like Joe O'Brien, the men's Debate Coach at Penn State, and Bob Newman (a Robert Redford look-alike) and Matty Ann Ditty, both of the University of Pittsburg, with their strong debate program. I was even briefly an officer in the Debate Association of Pennsylvania Colleges.

Back to Bethlehem, where Jean was teaching one of the lower grades with a lady named Emma Jordan, who had two sons and a daughter. More serendipity — fast-forward thirty years and I found an adult Carl Jordan knocking on the door in my carport, asking me if we could watch Danny and Timmy while he and his wife Ellen went house hunting. It's always a little odd when you see an adult you knew as a child, so many years later.

After the Freshleys left Pennsylvania, we ventured South, to the home of the University of Georgia, Athens, "The Classic City," where I still reside. In between tennis matches and raising a family, I taught Speech Communication at UGA for the remainder of my career, thoroughly enjoying the comforts of life "down South."

I'll summarize my career a little bit here, and I promise I'll just hit the highlights and keep it short. As a Speech professor, I taught thousands of students to keep their pronouncements pithy and to the point, so I should practice what I preached.

I was awarded a Fulbright Grant (Teaching Fellowship) in 1958 to teach in that "other" Athens. My time in Greece was an experience I'll always cherish. The fellowship lasted a full year, so I brought the family along. My son Phil was still very young, and his only real memory

VU Faculty Member To Teach In Greece

Dwight L. Freshley, assistant professor of speech at Vanderbilt University, will leave in September for a year in Athens, Greece, where he will teach in the college supported by the United States Educational Foundation.

Awarded a Fulbright grant for next year, he will direct speech activities, develop a forensic program and be in charge of the chapel programs and English clubs there in addition to teaching.

Before leaving for Athens, Prof. Freshley will attend a seminar on the teaching of English at the University of Michigan this summer. Mrs. Freshley and their son will accompany him.

Coming to Vanderbilt in 1955 from Ohio State University, Freshley teaches speech courses and directs forensics. He is a native of Homeworth, Ohio, and holds a Ph.D from Ohio State. A graduate of North Central College, Naperville, Ill., he also has an M.A. degree from Northwestern University.

Fulbright grants are made by the Board of Foreign Scholarships, whose members are appointed by the President of the United States. Under the Fulbright Act teachers now are being sent to more than 25 countries.

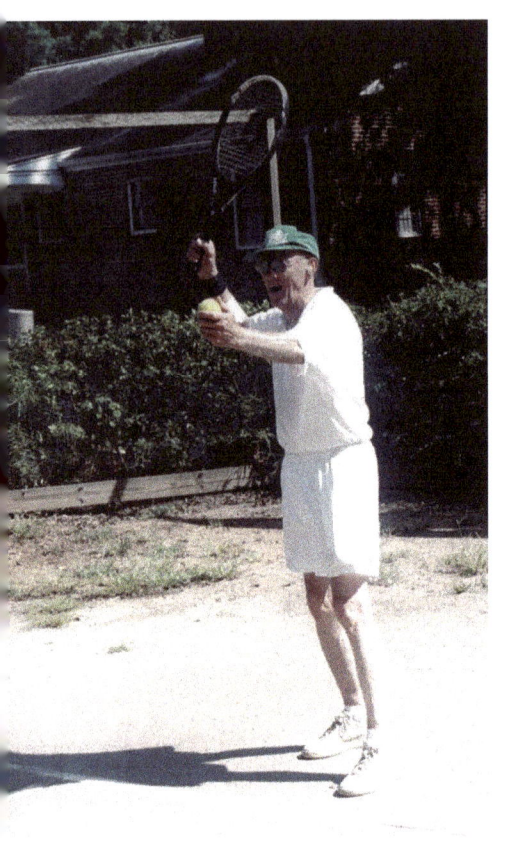

of that year was chasing little Mediterranean lizards over and around the crumbling monument to early democratic society, The Parthenon. Boys will be boys, even when they're growing up in the cradle of Western civilization. I vividly recall the small plaque next to the altar which read, "Please do not leave money on the altar. Children will steal it and we will be the cause of their sin."

From 1970 until 1973, I was the editor of the Southern Speech Journal, an outlet for regional scholars to publish their efforts, helping to preserve and study the nuances of our renowned and eclectic Southern speech history. As a native Midwesterner who never planned to move South, but loved it once I did, this Yankee took particular pride in Southern speech, co-authoring five textbooks on speech (analysis, communications, pretty much every aspect of speech) and had at least twenty articles published that I know of. Probably more.

In 1989, as the Berlin Wall was crumbling, I was given a Presidential Award for Distinguished Service for my work as the president of the Georgia Mental Health Association. I was the president of the Georgia Mental Health Association, having been plunged into that subculture because of the mental condition of my son. He showed me firsthand the variety that God grants the world. Jean and I threw ourselves into the betterment of the lives of local mentally ill people. I hope I helped make their lives a little better. Mental illness is a large and largely misunderstood problem, one that we've yet to even come close to solving.

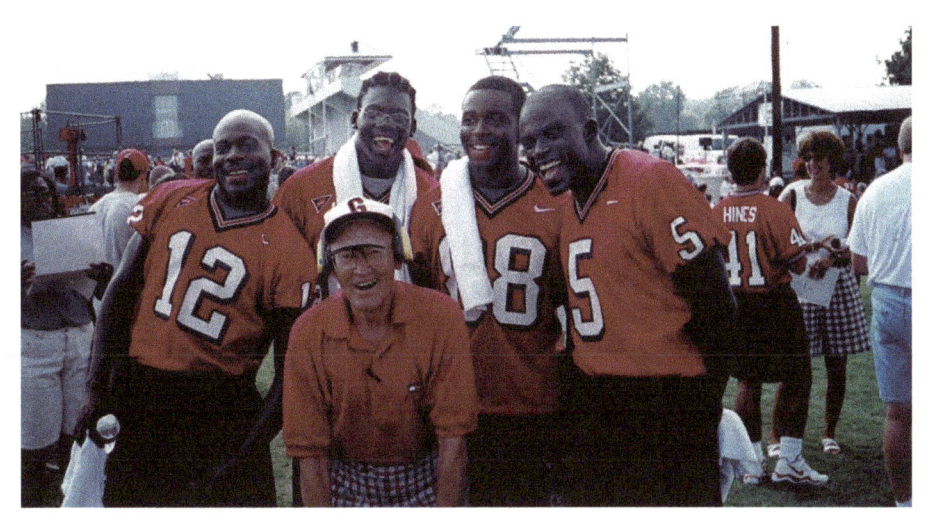

In the 1990's, I retired and immediately went to China to teach as a Visiting Professor at Renmin University (The People's University), as one does. Every year since 1995, the Southern States Communication Association has presented the Dwight L. Freshley Outstanding New Teacher Award to a bright young educator recently set out on his or her path. It makes me feel good to know that this award helps young people who want to study and teach Speech Communications to even younger people, as I did.

One of my missions in life has been to eradicate prejudice, to change the minds of people with ingrained hatred, to make this world a kinder, more understanding, infinitely more tolerant place to live. I like to think I have fulfilled this mission, at least in some small way.

I've already said that Talmadge Terrace, my current residence, has been a good fit for me. Nutritious, delicious cuisine, harmonious living, interesting neighbors, a king-sized bed, a cozy L-shaped room, and a 46-inch TV. What a life!

Addenda

EXTENSION STORY

Ellen Jordan was the top in her law class at Columbia. Soon after arriving to UGA, to become the Assistant Dean of the University of Georgia's Law School, she was asked to be Dean of the University of California, Davis Law School. She had only been out in the Golden State only a few months when she was diagnosed with ovarian cancer. Sadly, she had not been there long enough to earn enough health coverage to get through the medical procedures. To the everlasting credit of the University of Georgia (UGA), they hired her to teach that fall quarter. Ellen died in March or April. At her memorial service at UGA, her son Danny, who was at the time playing with the Cleveland Symphony, came down, bringing his own accompanist. It was one of the most beautiful and impressive services I've ever attended.

UP TO DATE IRONY — Carl Jordan later proceeded to buy my house! And two weeks ago he took me to two concerts at Hodgson Hall: 1) a trombone, piano and saxophone recital in the small concert hall, and then 2) We moved into the main auditorium for the largest assembly I've ever seen. Great venue.

MEMORABLE CLASSMATES FROM HOMEWORTH:

---Jack Peterson – son of owners of the Greek restaurant. We still keep in touch when I go back for family reunions. I spent one of my first overnights at his place. I also touch base with Ellen Staffer and her hubby Ray.

—Lyle— overcame tuberculosis, with a dragging right leg, played a "mean" game of ping pong and tennis. He remained a friend for life. I still keep in touch with his daughter, Jenny, who worked in the mayor's office. Her sister, Lois Anne was sweet on Paul.

—Al Cohen – fellow Esquirer/double-dater.

SERENDIPITIES FROM MY TIME IN THE MILITARY:

1) President Harry Truman's nephew came through my gates when I was in charge of checking homebound troops onto their ships, right after VE Day.

2) Warren Mockerman from my tiny hometown of Homeworth, Ohio was on that same list. He lived on the other side of town.

   I've always had music in my life. A big thing in Ohio was for high school orchestras to inaugurate the Akron Rubber Bowl (Goodyear, Goodrich, Firestone – Ohio's big on rubber.). I played the snare drum in the marching band and tympani in the concert orchestra. Earl Beach was our conductor. I was born into a musical family, with a piano teacher for a big sister and a spot on-stage with the family band awaiting my reaching adolescence. I'm still a music guy. Some things never change.

THE LYRICS TO A SONG I WROTE

(and almost was able to sell to a record company):

WANTED

Search every city,
Comb every town,
Look o'er the countryside
Up and down.
Take care
Everywhere,
She's WANTED.
Armed with a dangerous smile, she'll resist,
But she'll surrender when she's kissed.
Beware
I must be there.
The crime she committed was unforgivable,
She stole my heart away.
And that made my life unlivable,
But I'll find her
Come what may.
WANTED
I'd give a fortune for her return,
But if she comes back
It's my concern
That I must be WANTED, too.

76

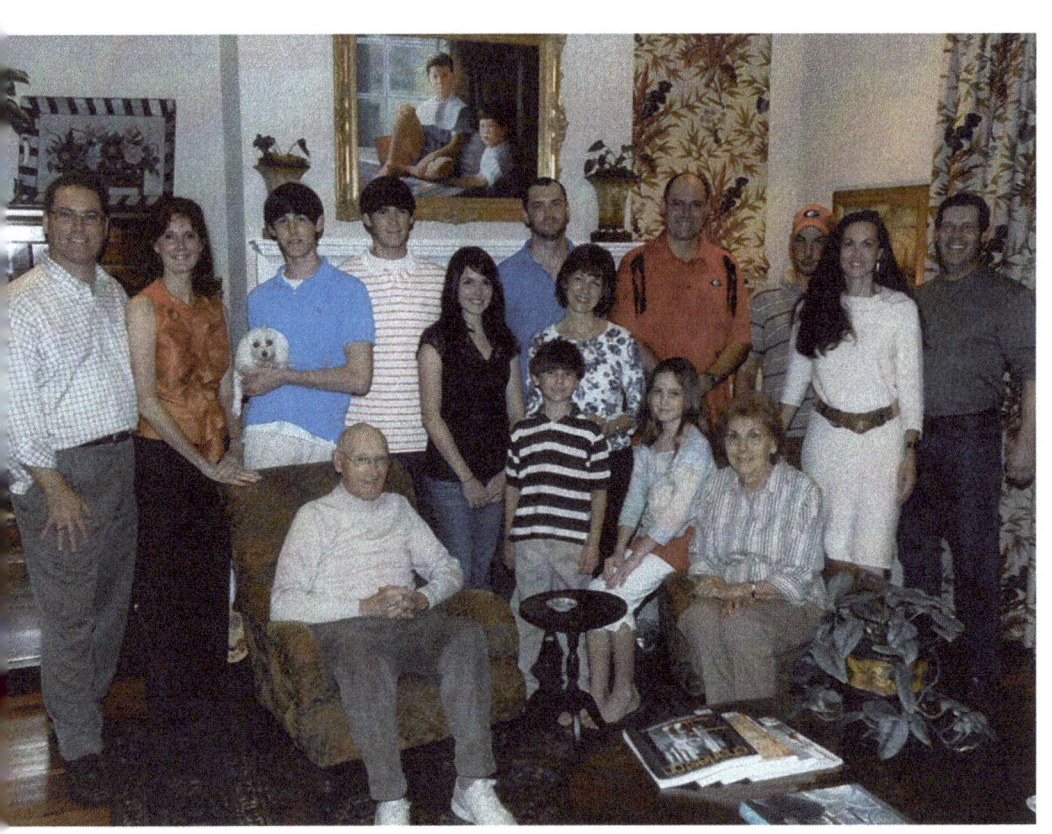

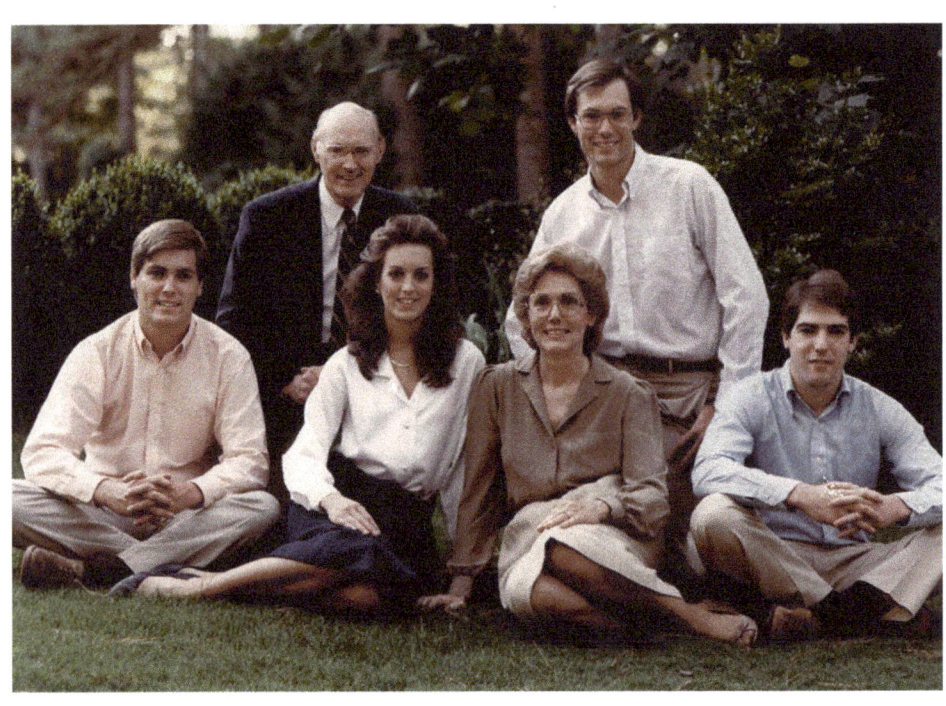

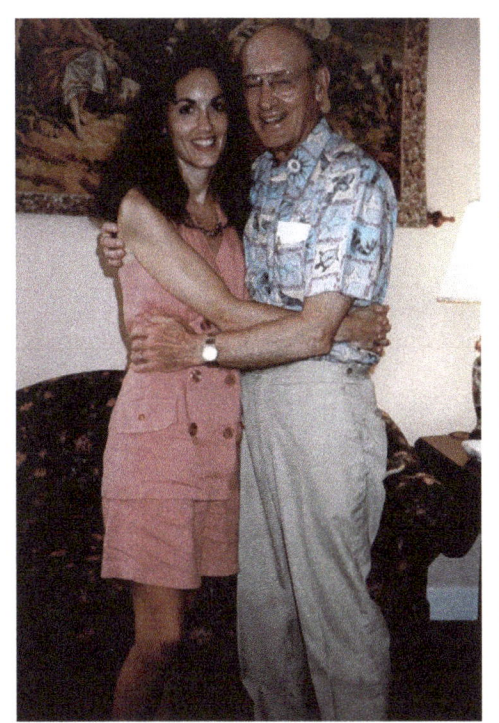

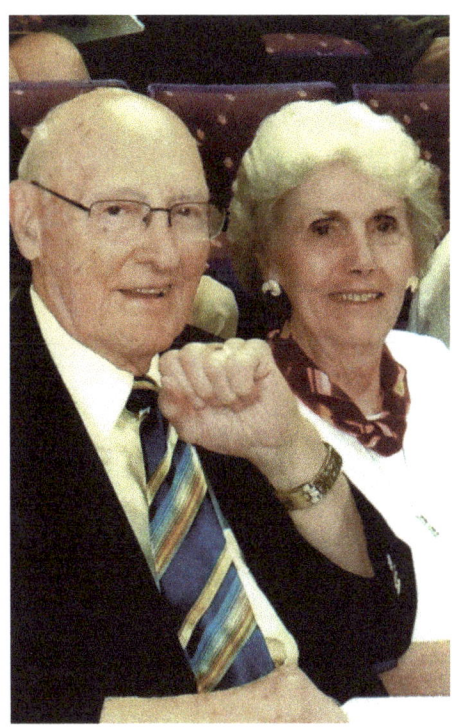

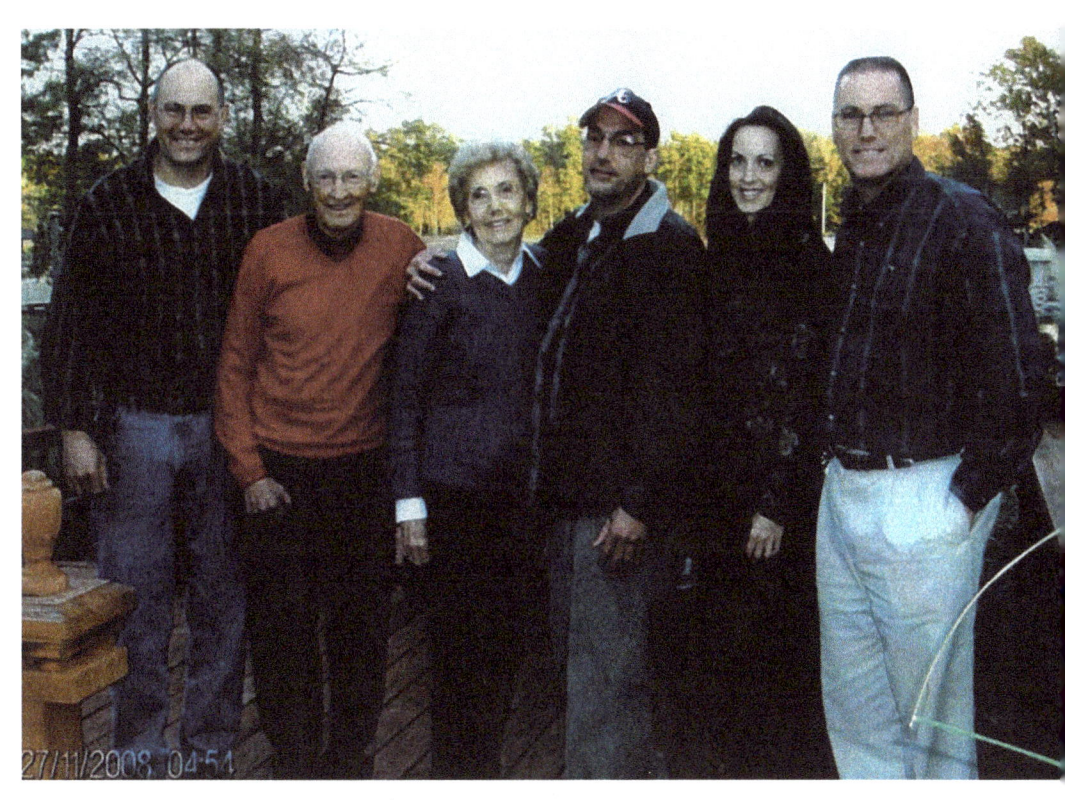

Raised on a dairy farm in Homeworth, Ohio, Dwight (Dee) Freshley, the youngest of seven children enlisted in World War II, served in Europe in the famous D-Day effort, and went to college on the GI Bill. He excelled in high school and college in both academics and student politics, becoming class president in both high school and college. With a doctorate from Ohio State, Dee served as a Professor and debate coach at Vanderbilt University, and advanced his career as a Speech Professor at the University of Georgia, serving for over a decade as Department Head. He worked until his 70's and retired as Professor Emeritus. Sweethearts at North Central University, Dee married Jean Reinhart. They raised four children in Nashville, Tennessee and Athens, GA, imbuing them with the values of two strong families learned over six decades.